Get the Most
——— out of ———
Motherhood

A Hot Mess to Mindful Mom Parenting Guide

Ali Katz

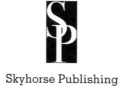

Skyhorse Publishing

This book is dedicated to:

Mark, Adam, and Dylan

You three are my everything.

Contents

Introduction

If you read my first book, you know me pretty well, and it means the world to me that you came back for more! If this is your first experience reading one of my books, welcome!

I am a real mom, just like you, trying hard to raise the best kids I can and to become the best version of myself in the process. Constantly wishing for parenting do-overs got old really fast, and I knew things had to change. I am also here to tell you that this stuff really works! These tips and tools can change your parenting and, by default, your life.

You are not alone. Every mom, myself included, feels clueless and lost at times. I have spent many sleepless nights guilt-ridden after yelling at my kids. You too? It often seems like raising kids is easier for everyone else. I don't believe that's true; I think that some people are simply more honest about the struggle.

This book is for moms who:

- Want to solidify a close relationship with their kids before they hit the teen years.

- Have kids that are between the ages of five and twelve.
- Are looking to stay ahead of consequences and not feel like they are punishing their kids all the time.
- Want to stop fighting with their kids and constantly feeling frustrated.
- Want to create balance between being "Mom" and being *You*.
- Want to actually enjoy raising their kids.
- Want to connect with their kids on a deeper level and truly bond.
- Just want to stop yelling all the time!

We only have so much time before our kids are full-fledged teenagers who will attempt to pull away from us faster than we can imagine. The years from five to twelve are incredibly formative ones, and are our chance to create a relationship with our kids that is built on mutual trust, communication, and respect. I have always believed that parents should act like parents and not try to be friends with their kids—I had a different experience growing up, and it never felt right to me. When I had my own children, I knew I wanted to do things differently.

I have found that strong boundaries, clear expectations, and a ton of love create an environment in my home that feels good to everyone involved. My kids know how much we love them, but also that we won't stand for disrespect.

You will immediately notice when you start reading that I am pretty much an open book (pun intended!) and that I share my ideas by sharing my personal experiences. I don't pretend for one second that I am perfect—as a mom or a person—but I have spent the last few years becoming stronger in both areas. I don't have grandiose ideas that one can actually obtain perfection in any area of one's life, but my philosophy is this: if my keen awareness helps me to figure out what doesn't work, I can choose differently the next time I am in a similar situation, with hopefully better results. This is one of the ways that I have gone from "hot mess" to "mindful mom." I am hyperaware of myself these days.

I am passionate about helping other women transform their lives as I have. It has taken soul-searching, trial and error, and a few misses along with many hits, but because I am at it day in and day out, I have tons of ideas to share, and it is my passion and life's purpose to share them.

I am a certified self-care and mindful parenting coach, a meditation expert, a speaker, and obviously, an author. I have two spirited boys and tons of street cred. I practice what I preach, even though admittedly some days go better than others, but I always try my best and aim to constantly grow both in parenthood and life. Some days it feels like I teach what I've learned, and other days I teach what I *need* to learn.

There are three unique sections in this book to help you achieve your goal of becoming a more mindful mom and the very best version of yourself:

Mindful Mom Mindset covers bringing your very best self to your parenting.

Mindful Mom Methods offers suggestions for creating structure in your home.

Mindful Mom Moments offers ideas and techniques for bonding with your kids.

I am excited and honored to share my ideas, tactics, and tips with you. I get pretty personal and basically invite you into my home life and into my family, so we must be friends already!

Don't wait to make the changes in yourself and your home that you have been thinking about forever. Don't wait because you think it is too hard or it won't work. Get started today and become the best mom you can be. You'll be doing the work, but I'll be guiding you every step of the way, and I can guarantee it will be some of the most rewarding work you will do in your life.

I have personally utilized every tactic that I share, and I teach them to all of my clients with amazing results. My clients tell me that the entire environment in their home changes with these tools, and you can have the same result, too. I am so excited for you to start your Mindful Mom journey!

Get cozy, savor a mug of your favorite tea (mine is a chai tea misto with unsweetened vanilla almond milk, a dash of cinnamon, and a bit of raw honey), and let's jump in.

SECTION 1

Mindful Mom Mindset

As moms, we have the unique ability—and responsibility—to set the tone in our homes. I don't know about you, but if I am having an "off day," everyone in my house can tell. My energy affects everyone around me, for better or worse.

Over the past few years, because I have really focused on self-care and mindfulness, the feeling in my home has changed, literally because I have changed. Before my journey began, I often felt exhausted, overwhelmed, and depleted, and that was the version of me that my family got.

I won't pretend that I don't ever have off days anymore, but they are fewer and farther between because I take the time to fill my own cup, nurture myself, and admit when something isn't working and needs to change. I no longer just throw my hands up in the air ready to give up when something doesn't work. Now I have the tools I need to make the appropriate adjustments so I feel like "me," and the energy in my home is the best it can be. My awareness and willingness to try new things has led to creative solutions that I now feel passionate about sharing with other moms.

When we are able to bring our best self to our parenting, we enjoy being a parent more. I know that sounds like a simple concept, but it takes dedication and some trial and error to make it happen. There are moments of parenting that feel more challenging, and others that seem to glide by with ease and grace, and in those we see and feel how our effort and commitment pay off. That is until the next challenging time, when we recommit and double down our efforts.

These tools I share aren't one-and-done ideas. They are simple steps you can take to create new habits for yourself and your family that seamlessly fit into your life. The ideas I share are proof that small changes and tweaks can have a major impact when we use them consistently. They aren't rocket science, either! I have so many clients that ask me during our sessions, "Why didn't I think of that?!" My philosophy hasn't changed in years . . . simple works.

The lessons in the following Mindful Mom Mindset section are full of tools and ideas to help you step into the most authentic version of yourself. The one full of love, presence, gratitude, and peace. If you are rolling your eyes right now, STOP! That is who you are! At our core, we are pure love and peace, but the craziness of life often gets in the way of accessing it.

The ideas I share will help you to slow down a bit. They will guide you to feel the power that your presence has. And they will just make you feel good! Your relationship with your kids will improve as your relationship with yourself improves. So let's get started!

1

What Is Mindful Parenting?

Mindfulness is more than a buzzword!

"Parenting is the easiest thing in the world to have an opinion about, but the hardest thing in the world to do."

—MATT WALSH

The best way to illustrate what mindful parenting is . . . is to show you what it isn't. Here goes—my all-time parenting low!

My son was about five years old at the time, and he was driving me nuts. Five years later, I can't remember exactly what he was doing, which probably goes to show just what my tolerance level was at the time. He didn't light the house on fire, strip naked and pee on the floor, or smack me across the face. He most likely wasn't listening or was being mean to his brother. Regardless, I was having a very difficult time holding it together. I grabbed his arm and squeezed really, really hard. He cried, "Mommy, you are hurting me!" and I hissed, "On purpose."

This was the only time I have ever hurt one of my children physically, and I have worked hard to forgive myself for that. In the past

few years as I have transformed as a person and a parent, I have found compassion for the lost mom that I was. I didn't have the tools at the time that I needed to parent successfully. It's almost like I was floating down a river on a raft with no paddle. When the water was calm, the sun was shining, and my kids were behaving like perfect angels, we were great. But when the storm clouds came and brought a bit of wind and my kids acted, well, like kids, I had a hard time holding it together.

Nobody filled me in and explained that I needed tools, or gave me tools for that matter, to help with the stress of raising kids. It still amazes me that you need a license to drive a car, but anyone can be a parent. How is there no training class, or some sort of required reading at least?

Since then I have found a better way to parent and to live. As I continue to incorporate mindfulness into my life, I flourish, and so does my relationship with my children.

My personal transformation has allowed me to:

- Find calm in the chaos of raising my family
- Trust myself more and connect to my instincts and abilities
- Develop my confidence as a parent
- Remain calm and centered when all hell breaks loose
- Enjoy my life like never before

"Mindfulness" is a big buzzword these days. You can hardly open a magazine or watch a news show without it coming up. My definition of mindfulness is being fully engaged in every experience without judging it.

After both flailing and succeeding as a parent, I realized it was imperative to bring mindfulness into parenting my kids. For one,

I realized that I don't get a do-over. I wanted to be in the moment and enjoy raising my kids *now.* Even though some days crawl by, the months and years seem to fly at lightning speed. They will be out of my home and creating their own before I know it, so I want to be in the moment with my kids, sharing experiences and strengthening my relationship with them while I still have the chance.

To break it down to the most basic level, being a mindful mom to me means that I am not just getting through the days, but I am actually enjoying them and being engaged in them. I am not just going through the motions. I am thriving in my day-to-day life. The rest of this book is filled with ideas for how to make this a reality in your life, too.

So what keeps us from being mindful? So many things can contribute to this epidemic, but a few off the top of my head are judgment, comparison, and fear.

Unfortunately, judgment is prevalent in just about every area of parenting, and it keeps us from being in the present moment with our families. We judge ourselves, we judge other parents, and we judge our own kids and their friends, even if we don't mean to.

Over the years I've felt guilty and second-guessed nearly every major parenting decision, but I finally understand that it has kept me from becoming the kind of mom I want to be. Staying stuck in judgment inhibits me from actually growing. I can finally understand that I am so hard on myself because of my own insecurity and fear of making mistakes.

When a situation triggers sadness, judgment, comparison, or fear, I realize that I am definitely not in the present moment any longer. This is something really cool that I actually learned through my meditation studies: when we are feeling sad or depressed, our attention is in the past, and when we are feeling stressed or agitated,

our attention is in the future. We feel peaceful and content when our attention is in the present moment. It is my job to notice what is triggering me, why I can't let it go, and where it is carrying my attention. By releasing the urge to let this trigger carry me away to "no mom's land," I can stay focused on the present moment and what is really happening right now.

Everyone has a unique tolerance level, and different situations may trigger some moms and not others, but a few common provocations are:

- A nasty comment from another mom
- Second-guessing a parenting decision
- Worrying about what our kids are doing because of what we did at their age
- Kids who are not listening or are being disrespectful

"No mom's land" is a place in the mind far, far away from the present moment. It is where insecurity, judgment, and worry live. It isn't a fun place at all, so it's easy to wonder why we spend so much time there.

The shuttle back from this dark and barren land full of time-outs and desperation runs on awareness. When we are aware that we are triggered, and are spending time in the past or worrying about the future, it is our awareness that brings us back to the present moment.

Mindfulness can be achieved in many ways, for example, by paying attention to our breath, the sensations of our body, or by saying an affirmation. We basically want to redirect our attention back to the present moment. (Promise there will be more on how to actually do this is in later chapters, so stay tuned!)

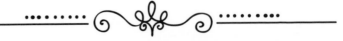

You know that feeling of being at your child's sporting event, and even though your eyes are technically on the field, your mind is somewhere else? Even though you were physically at the game, you pretty much missed it. Well, there isn't a do-over for that.

When we are mindful we can find more joy and fulfillment in our lives. We are more engaged with our families and more connected to ourselves. Mindfulness is a game changer. The more mindful I am as a person and a parent, the more I feel like I am really living.

This isn't to say that I wear rose-colored glasses all the time. I don't skip around with a big smile pasted on my face every minute of the day thinking everything is sunshine and roses. Yes, I find joy in more ways, and I feel grateful all day long, but I still experience pain, stress, and discomfort, just like everyone else. I simply recover faster because I have the tools to bring myself back to the present moment. I seem to learn my lessons faster and grow from them at a quicker pace than I used to.

Living a mindful life takes commitment, awareness, and dedication to your practice even when you want to pull your hair out as you magic-eraser crayon off the wall. You are never finished being mindful. This is how I plan to live the rest of my life; it's an exciting surprise to see where it takes me. If I have made this much progress recently, where will I be in five, ten, or twenty years? I am going to be pretty freaking awesome!

2

Crowding Out

Release negative mind chatter related to your parenting

"You need to learn how to select your thoughts just the same way you select your clothes every day. This is a power you cultivate."

—ELIZABETH GILBERT

When I think of "crowding out," I immediately think of a diet book I once read. It described the concept of crowding out as the key to eating only healthy foods. The premise is that if you have enough servings of fruits, veggies, and protein in a day you'll be so full that you won't have room for junk. You basically crowd out the junk from your diet.

This actually made tons of sense to me and flipped on a lightbulb in my mind. If I can do this with food, can I do this with my thoughts?

In my meditation teacher training, I learned so much about how our emotions can give us big-time clues as to where our thoughts and attention are.

If we feel sadness or feelings of depression, our mind is in the past.

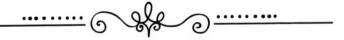

If we feel anxiety or worry, our mind is in the future.

If we feel peace, our mind is in the present.

Basically, we just need to keep our minds in the present all the time, so no more ruminating about the past or worrying about the future. Easier said than done!

What I have noticed about myself, and most of my clients, is that we each tend to lean toward one end of the spectrum by spending most of our time ruminating or worrying. There are a few people split down the middle, but most are not.

I am more of a ruminator. If I could have the hours back that I spent reliving conversations in my head and beating myself up over silly comments I made, I just may have the amount of hours it takes to go to medical school, law school, or have written many, many books by now. It is crazy to think about how many hours and how much energy I have wasted—but then I realize that I'm just ruminating more!

I have taken it so far as to sit up all night thinking about a comment I made that I blew up in my head as something that offended the other person or hurt their feelings. I imagined them sitting up all night thinking what an insensitive idiot I was—so much so that I even called the next morning to apologize. Of course, they didn't even remember what I was talking about! Time showed me that it was incredibly egocentric of me, and that most people aren't paying that much attention to what I do or say because they have a ton going on in their own lives.

What I have learned during my transformation is that nothing I do or say is going to change the past, and that is okay. I can't wish a do-over into existence or crawl under a rock until the other person forgets what I said. What I can do is change my energy around the situation.

There is a zen proverb I especially love that holds deep meaning for many of my clients as well: "let go or be dragged." We have to let go of the past or it will drag us down.

For every moment that I spend beating myself up about something I cannot change, I lose a moment of joy. I steal from myself because I am robbing myself of the present moment.

Realizing this allowed me to transition from a victim mentality to an empowered one. By returning to the present moment in times when I would ordinarily be ruminating, I increase my joy and happiness. But how do I do it? There are a few ways, and I am ready to share away!

The first is that I practice bringing my thoughts back to the present by connecting with my breath and body, and doing what I call a "one-minute meditation." One-minute meditations are amazing to use in many situations, such as:

When you are ruminating or future-tripping

Whenever I notice that I am in the past or the future, it is time to re-center myself.

Whenever you feel stressed or triggered

This can be in a meeting, as tension mounts with a family member or friend, or whenever you feel overwhelmed or exhausted.

Transition times

I am a firm believer that we all jump from one role to the next without giving ourselves a second to breathe and prepare.

Think about these transitions:

- Mom to work
- Work to mom
- Getting ready to pick up the kids in the carpool lane
- Heading into a volunteer commitment at school
- Working at your computer before entering a meeting

Taking one minute to regroup and switch gears can set the tone and prepare you for clear thinking, patience, and productivity.

When you are trying to fall asleep

It can feel hard to let go of your day. One minute of meditation can help to calm your nervous system and get you one step closer to a good night's sleep.

Downtime at a traffic light or in line at a store

Any time that used to be considered wasted can now be put to very good use. You can turn any minute into a mindful one. Don't mindlessly reach for your phone; reach for your breath instead.

When your kids are frustrating you

One of the biggest benefits of meditation is that it teaches you to be less reactive and more responsive. I notice this the most with my kids. Instead of yelling at them and then feeling guilty for hours afterward, I take a minute to breathe and then respond to them in a thoughtful manner that makes me feel like the calm, cool, and collected mom I thought I'd never be.

I've also begun to understand that I have a wonderful opportunity to learn from the past. Every situation has something to teach us. Some experiences are fun and enjoyable, and others are uncomfortable, messy, and decidedly un-fun to go through. However, each offers us a lesson and an opportunity to grow as a person.

I firmly believe that the Universe doesn't do anything *to* us, only *for* us. Everything we go through serves a purpose and leads us to become the best version of ourselves. This realization allowed me to see the places I messed up as amazing assignments and chances to grow, or cosmic redirections, if you will.

Fortunately, because I like to look at the glass as half full, we can do better when we know better. Making mistakes and saying things I regret has taught me to slow down, to think before I speak, and to read situations better. I'm not saying I never make comments I regret, but they are fewer and further between, thank goodness. I am also quicker at learning the lesson from them and offering myself comfort and understanding afterward.

I also show myself compassion in the moment by making decisions that feel right for me and help me to honor what I need. I've realized that I need to take time to consider my own feelings as well as other people's, and this is much easier to do if I slow down a bit. For example, saying "yes" when I really want to say "no," and then regretting it became a lesson to honor my desires. Feeling overwhelmed and overscheduled became a reality check for maintaining balance and joy in my life.

A concept that I truly believe in, and that I teach many of my clients about, is that we can make choices moment by moment to shift our energy and come back to the present.

Think about days when you totally splurge at breakfast on that big stack of pancakes covered in butter and syrup, and then you pig

out at lunch. Maybe you think, "Oh well, may as well finish off the day with that burger and fries for dinner." But we don't have to do that! We can change direction, have a salad for dinner, and feel so much better. We can do that with our energy, too!

If we are having a difficult day and beating ourselves up about it, we don't have to continue on that path. We can change direction at any time by deciding that we want to bring a fresh perspective and better energy to the next moment. Realizing that this is in our control is extremely empowering. If we want to change the course of our day, we simply need to take action to make that happen. A large shift may be required, like skipping our errands because we know that we need some down time, rescheduling a meeting if possible, or telling the kids to get dressed quickly because a fun family outing is just what is needed to turn the day around.

Not all shifts need to be that grandiose, however. Sometimes taking one minute for yourself to regroup is just what the Universe ordered. Your breath should really be your BFF in times like these. One-minute meditations are my standard go-to, day in and day out. Nothing shifts my energy as quickly and efficiently.

A few of my favorite one-minute meditations are:

Matching my inhale and exhale for one minute

My favorite way to do this is to take a comfortable inhale and silently count to three in my head as I breathe in. Then I match that count of three in my head as I exhale.

Doing a one-minute body scan

If your body is tense, your mind doesn't have a chance of relaxing. Hit the highlights such as your face, your shoulders, your chest, and

your belly, and be sure that each area is relaxed. If you notice tension in any area, breathe into it and feel that body part relax.

Paying attention to my senses

This is another amazing tool for getting out of your head and into your body in order to connect with the present moment. In one minute, notice what you can see, hear, smell, touch, and taste. It is virtually impossible for your mind to wander during this exercise. Try it!

Peace Begins With Me

This simple Kundalini meditation of touching your fingertips together, that I learned from one of my mentors, Gabby Bernstein, is one of my favorites and is a great one to teach your kids as well. It's also my husband's favorite one-minute meditation. He has taught it to everyone at work, which I love!

Touch the tips of your thumb and forefinger together and silently say PEACE.

Touch the tips of your thumb and middle finger together and silently say BEGINS.

Touch the tips of your thumb and ring finger together and silently say WITH.

Touch the tips of your thumb and pinky together and silently say ME.

Counting my breaths for one minute

You can get yourself out of the crazy stories in your head with this technique as well. Inhale and silently think *one.* Exhale and think

two. Inhale and think three. Exhale and think four . . . Continue up to ten and then start over.

Belly Breathing

We may think we are taking deep breaths, but by breathing into our clavicle area only, we are actually activating our fight-or-flight response, also known as the stress response. Someone is doing this when you see them take a deep breath and they lift their shoulders. We see kids do this often as well.

We need to fill our entire clavicle, chest, and belly areas with fresh oxygen. We can do this by belly breathing.

Put your hand on your belly under your belly button. Breathe in like you are blowing up a balloon in your belly. Then exhale and let all the air out of your balloon.

I use these tools day in and day out to refocus my attention when it is stuck in an unproductive place. They especially came in handy when I attended a ten-day silent Vipassana retreat.

I read about Dan Harris's experience at a ten-day silent retreat a few years ago in his book *10% Happier*, and for some reason, as a pretty new meditator, I remember saying to myself, "I'll definitely do that one day."

Taking my experiences to the extreme is a definite personality trait. I am sure that a psychologist could go to town on this one! When I started running at thirty-five, I signed up for a half-marathon as motivation. During the race I saw the full marathoners continuing straight on the road to their finish, but I had to turn around to complete my half distance. I was burning inside, and in that moment I just knew that I would one day run a marathon. I wanted to be one of the people going further.

Once I got certified as a meditation teacher, I began to feel an inexplicable tug to sit for a ten-day silent meditation retreat, and I decided it was going to be my fortieth birthday present to myself. I felt that it would help take my practice to the next level, just like running a full marathon took my athleticism to another level. I felt ready and up for the challenge.

The overwhelming response I got from people when they found out I was going was "Why?" or "I don't get it!" I totally understand how crazy it seems to voluntarily disconnect from everything, not talk for ten days, and meditate for a hundred hours in that time. I really do. And I didn't even have a very good answer beyond, "I just need to do this." The truth is that I had no real expectations. I didn't know what would happen or how I would change; I simply felt a call, and I listened.

I didn't research or ask a million people about their experiences. Basically the only two words I've ever heard used to describe a ten-day sit are "transformational" and "excruciating." I didn't really need to hear more! I wanted to have no preconceived ideas or expectations.

Fortunately there is a Vipassana Meditation Center about four hours from Houston, so the trip seemed easy enough and I signed up six months in advance. Truthfully, in my heart I had committed even six months before that because I started turning down other retreat opportunities, and the reason I gave was that this was the year I was doing a ten-day silent retreat.

I had no clue what Vipassana was all about, but I felt pretty much game for anything having to do with meditation and any sort of experience that would level up my practice.

The weeks leading up to my departure, my nerves kicked in big time, but about a week or two before I left, they completely dissipated. I was so sure that this was the right next step for my personal

growth and development, as well as my meditation practice, and I had no doubts.

The packing was super easy! Ten sets of sweatpants and sweat-shirts, face wash, lotion, shampoo, a comb, comfy socks, and Uggs, and that was basically it. I was going to have ten days with no makeup, no blow-dryer, no fixing snacks, no cooking dinner, no technology, and no access to the outside world beyond the retreat boundaries. I was excited and terrified. I left in the middle of my obsessive Netflix binge of *Parenthood*, right before Christina had her baby, and honestly the hardest part was that I would have to wait till I got home to see the baby be born.

Saying goodbye to Mark and the boys was hard. I put Adam to bed crying the night before and did everything I could think of to prepare. Mark had a five-page list of instructions, and the boys had a letter to read from me every day and a video of me saying good-night to watch before bed each night. Mark was basically a superhero and completely took over my household duties in addition to work. My mother-in-law pitched in big time, and I had great friends that helped a ton. I was beyond blessed to have this support system. It was the only way that I could go.

Heading to the retreat center was an adventure in itself as I navi-gated winding country roads. It was only the second time that I had driven more than an hour myself, so it already felt like a new level of independence was being reached.

I spent the car ride on the phone saying goodbye to my family and close friends, and as I pulled in I felt ready for my experience to begin, yet it felt surreal at the same time. I met two sweet girls, the only two names I would know for ten days, and we walked the grounds and unloaded our cars together.

The time quickly came to turn in my car keys, wallet, and cell phone, unpack, and get ready for orientation. I called Mark for one last quick goodbye, and that was the moment that I began to panic. My voice cracked and I simply said one more "I love you" with a few tears in my eyes, and then quickly hung up before I changed my mind about the whole thing altogether.

It felt oddly freeing to turn in my car keys, wallet, and phone, but as I walked into my small private room to unpack I will now admit that I threw up in my mouth. The reality of what I was about to do, and how disconnected from my family I was going to be, hit me like a tidal wave. The only way to calm myself down was to breathe and remember that I had chosen this. I had to believe that I was in the right place, at the right time, doing just what I needed to do for myself. I simply had to.

Since there were no distractions from my thoughts for ten days straight, I was front and center for a few that showed me how much work I still had to do. I compared myself to others, I judged myself and my progress, and I internally lost my shit when the people around me cracked their knuckles incessantly (which sends me over the edge). No matter how much work I do on myself, there will always be more! But I did learn a ton about myself, and here are a few of the standout lessons for me:

Some days you have to make your own chai!

On Day Two there was the most amazing chai served with breakfast. I mean, divine. It was second only to the chai at ChocolaTree in Sedona, and that is saying a lot. If you ever make it to Sedona, you must go! I woke up on Day Four dreaming of the homemade chai. I was lying in bed at 4:00 a.m. after the gong woke me up, willing it to be at breakfast. It wasn't, and I was a little sad when I walked in, but

I realized that I had a choice. I could be disappointed that nobody made me chai, or I could grab a chai tea bag, milk, honey, and cinnamon, and create a version for myself. I admit, it wasn't as delicious as Day Two's, but it was good enough, and I had chai.

Chai became a metaphor for me that morning. I can wait around for things to show up in life, or I can make them happen. In the future, when I feel disappointed about something not happening for me, I will remember this chai and figure out another way to get as close as I can.

Show up for yourself!

I started hearing the gong they woke us up with and used to call us to meditations throughout the day, even when it wasn't ringing. I heard it in the middle of the night when I rolled over. I heard it while I was walking around the pond. I contemplated if I could get PTSD from the gong.

I have to do things all the time that I don't want to do, like going to the grocery store, packing lunch for the millionth time, and doing dishes for what seems like every second of the day. However, in those cases there are people counting on me. Am I going to look at my kids and tell them, "Sorry guys, you don't have lunch today. I didn't feel like making it"? Nope, but the difference is this experience was just for me.

I wasn't on a spa vacation. People hear the words "silent retreat" and assume it's relaxing, but I worked so damn hard.

I found out how far I was willing to go for myself. There were plenty of times that I had to remind myself that I wanted this. I am worth the work. I will go out on a limb for myself and do just what I think I can't do because I am that important in my own life. This was a ten-day commitment to myself, and there was no way I was quitting. I found out just what I am capable of.

Some moments were torture, and some were among the proudest of my life. At times I wanted to run, but I couldn't leave myself. I had to be my biggest support system and my own best friend. This was an extreme, I give you that. We can be our own best friend in many small ways in our day-to-day lives, and we should. But for some reason at this point in my life I needed to not only be there for my family, friends, and clients, I needed to see how far I would go for *me*. That was the pull I felt, and what I couldn't explain until I actually accomplished it.

I know this experience will make me a better wife, mom, coach, teacher, friend, daughter, sister, and most of all, *me*. I now know just how strong I am. I feel like I am my own best friend, and what I get from others is like the icing on the cake.

You are never done

You may not like what you see when every thought is front and center, but you must love and accept yourself—and find compassion for yourself, too. I am not perfect, and it has never been more obvious than after ten days alone with my thoughts. To be honest, there were moments that I was shocked and disappointed by certain thoughts that I had while I was away. I thought I had gotten past some of the judgements and insecurities that surfaced. What I realized, though, is that my only choice is to try every day to be better, and to make progress. I am committed even more deeply to learn, grow, practice, release, try, do better, fail, recommit, practice more, and dig deep.

I did finally slow down

I stopped getting annoyed at the people walking slowly in front of me and taking *forever* to mindfully wash their dishes when ten people

were standing in line behind them. I mean, what the heck else did I have to do?

Slowing down is a constant struggle in my everyday life. As a working mom trying to fit in clients, workouts, running errands, walking the dogs, and an occasional pedi and coffee with a friend all before carpool, homework, activities, and dinner, it isn't realistic to think I can maintain the speed of a slug all day long, but I have gained awareness and can feel the difference between warp speed and a comfortable pace. And let's not forget that my husband craves attention occasionally, too!

I am sitting down with the kids to have breakfast instead of running around the kitchen now, and it is so nice. Yes, it means getting downstairs ten minutes earlier in the morning, but I start the day with the kids feeling mindful and connected. Since your kids learn more from what you do than what you say, I need to walk the walk. I want them to enjoy all the precious moments of their lives, and I have the amazing opportunity to model that for them.

Usually when you want to give up, the good stuff is about to happen

I walked into our 2:30 p.m. meditation on Day Five with a sore ass and no desire to meditate. We were instructed by our teachers that three times a day from then on we would be doing "determination meditations," meaning we could no longer move or adjust. Our hands, feet, and closed eyes had to remain absolutely still.

I am a major fidgeter. I have never been perfectly still in my life and I was petrified. I really wanted to succeed, and you know what? I did! I was so incredibly proud. I literally shocked myself. I opened

my eyes afterward and broke into a huge smile. Out of the corner of my eye I saw the woman on the cushion next to me (I wouldn't learn her name for another five days) fist pump the air. I guess she did it for the first time, too!

Nature is absolutely amazing

The sights of nature were breathtaking. Since there were no distractions such as conversation or walking with my head bent toward my phone furiously typing, I was able to notice every fiery sunrise, pink and lavender sunset, stars that looked like polka dots in the sky, and the crystal-clear reflection on the pond. Since the retreat, I find myself still contemplating the beauty of nature on a daily basis. My kids have probably heard the phrase "God's paintbrush" a hundred times while I gaze at the sunset.

You always have to be willing to laugh at yourself

On the fourth day we were told that we were ready to learn the Vipassana technique. I was so confused because I thought we were doing the technique with the breathing exercises we were given on the first day. I thought I was totally rocking Vipassana, but it turns out that was just the warm up! The technique is layered, and new instructions came every two to three days with practice time in between. That is why the course had to be ten days—it took that much time to learn and practice. I got a good laugh at my expense. It was ignorance at its best!

During my re-entry I was bombarded with questions, but the one I was asked the most was, "Was it as hard as you thought it would be?"

If you had asked me on Day Three I would have told you no, but I can see with hindsight that I was in the honeymoon phase. I hadn't cried yet, and the days were going fairly quickly because everything was exciting and new and I was so happy to be on that journey.

In the early days I thought about the quote "Wherever you are, be all there" a lot. I was determined to be in the present moment and make the most of this opportunity to spend ten whole days focusing on my spiritual practice.

If you had asked me any time on Days Four through Eight, I would've told you that I now know what it feels like for time to completely stand still. The days seemed to take forever and I was riding out the emotional storms that kept creeping up, so it was the hardest part for me.

If you had asked me on Day Ten I would've told you that it wasn't that bad. You know how after being pregnant or running a marathon the good moments stand out much more than the difficult and painful ones? That is how I felt at the end.

In those ten days I felt every emotion on the spectrum of emotions.

I felt inspired.

I felt proud.

I felt wise.

I felt clueless.

I was judgmental of myself.

I was compassionate toward myself.

Meditations flew by; meditations dragged.

I could feel myself transforming.

I wondered if anything was happening at all.

I felt so sure of why I was there.

I had no clue why I was there.

I felt grateful.

I wanted to run.

I felt fulfilled.

I felt bored.

I felt lucky.

I felt crazy.

I had fun with myself.

I was sick of myself.

Now that it is over, I understand why the two most popular words people use when they reference ten-day retreats are "transformational" and "excruciating." I couldn't pick two better ones myself.

When I finally could talk to the other women who participated, all I wanted to know was what they did in their rooms when we had a few free minutes. Those ten- and twenty-minute periods were the hardest for me. I would have killed for a book to read! It turns out that how I occupied my time was pretty common—flossing my teeth, giving myself a foot rub, doing sit-ups and planks, and checking for zits. I mean, when was the last time you had ten minutes to give yourself a foot massage? Boredom made me pretty creative.

* * * * *

Our expectation of how things "should" be can ruin the actual experience if we let it. This could have easily have happened on my retreat, but I went in with a beginner's mind, meaning I had no preconceived ideas of what I wanted to happen. I have to practice this all the time with my kids, too.

Have you ever planned what you think is going to be the best day ever with your kids, and it turns to shit at the very end without fail? After a fun day at the zoo ending with a trip for ice cream

sundaes, your kids end up fighting in the car and the day ends with everyone in a foul mood.

We took our kids to Disneyland a few years ago and planned the most memorable day imaginable, complete with a character breakfast, a private guide, no lines, and front row seats for every show. Luckily, another family from Houston met us there and shared the expense, which was incredibly helpful. We gave our kids the royal treatment for two reasons which were both selfish on our part:

1. My husband and I don't love theme parks, so we wanted to get the entire park done in one day, and hit the beach for the rest of our California adventure.

2. We got to relax and enjoy the day, too. We let our guide handle every detail, and we followed her around like little ducklings. We never once glanced at a map, which is very lucky because my husband and I both have a horrible sense of direction, and we would have spent most of the day scrambling our way around the park and feeling frustrated, possibly with each other.

As we tucked our kids into bed after the fireworks display, we reviewed the day, talked about how grateful we all were, and asked the kids about their favorite parts of the day. We totally felt like parents of the freaking year and were excited to hear their responses! Was it riding the *Cars* ride three times in a row? Was it getting to fight Darth Vader in the *Star Wars* show on stage?

My little one (who was four at the time) told us it was a really great day, but it would have been *perfect* if he had gotten to meet Mickey Mouse. We went from feeling like parents of the year to total slackers! We went to Disneyland and never met Mickey. We saw him

in the parade but never gave him a hug or got his autograph. What had we been thinking—everyone knows you're supposed to meet Mickey! He found the one hole in our entire day! We felt like we went from "hero" to "zero."

We explained that Mickey is so busy all day at Disney, and sometimes it can be hard to find him, but we felt horrible! We spent half the night worrying and brainstorming about how to stalk Mickey quickly before we had to check out of our hotel in the morning.

My husband can pretty much make anything happen, so he somehow finagled and got us into Mickey's breakfast as we were rolling out of Disney the next morning. Someone had canceled last minute, just for us!

The more we try to go into situations with a beginner's mind, the better experience we will have, and this is also a lesson to teach our kids, and to help them practice. We had all had a great day, but it was nearly ruined as soon as we realized we had almost missed something that you're "supposed" to do in Disney.

We were able to turn this situation around and find Mickey, but there have been plenty of times that we haven't been able to make everything perfect for our kids, nor would it have served them. Life doesn't turn out exactly how we want it to all the time. However, different doesn't always mean bad; it just means different.

One of the biggest disappointments for our younger son was being held back in school. He was three at the time, so we didn't even think he would notice, but he cried practically every day after school for three years and told us numerous times that we ruined his life. It crushed me each and every time I heard it.

Once you decide to hold a kid back, there is really no turning back. My husband and I were steadfast in our belief that we did

the right thing by giving him a chance to be a leader and gain the confidence he lacked from being so young for his grade. Even so, it took him years to acclimate to his new grade, so much so that we contemplated switching schools just so he could have a fresh start. He finally became happier in his class, but his closest friends remain in the grade above him.

There were moments that we wondered if we really did ruin his life! This was something that we couldn't fix for him, instead we had to help him work through his emotions and frustrations. It was really hard, but we all learned from the experience.

Mark and I learned to trust our intuition and do what was right for our kid, even though it was the harder choice because he was happy socially in his old grade. Dylan learned that things in life aren't always exactly how we want them, but choosing to make the best of a situation, and having a good attitude about it, can change every-thing. Our attitude can make or break each of our life experiences, so we better pick a good one. When Dylan finally did stop worrying about the grade he thought he should be in and instead immersed himself a bit more in his new grade, his attitude about school did improve.

Learning to be flexible can make or break our stress levels. It is a gift we give to ourselves and one we should impart to our children. Life throws a ton of curveballs, and we have to roll with them. Some-times it's the idea in our head of exactly how we want things to be that holds us back. Occasionally the Universe has a better plan for us. I call this a cosmic redirection, and in these cases I have learned to surrender and trust.

3

Sunday Prep

Cook like a mad woman so your family can eat healthy all week long

"Spectacular achievement is always preceded by unspectacular preparation."
—ROBERT H. SCHULLER

I have been a petite person since the moment I made my debut on this earth. I was basically the runt of the litter, if twins count. I guess a tiny litter! My mom didn't know she was having twins—in fact, her third pregnancy was kind of a surprise, which I learned in my teens. The kind of surprise you refer to as a total blessing, of course.

Back in what seems like the olden days now, doctors only did ultrasounds if they thought something was wrong. It seemed as if my mom was having a normal, healthy pregnancy and was going to deliver one healthy baby. It turns out that my twin sister and I were head to toe in the womb, so it felt like one baby, and we had a simultaneous heartbeat, so it sounded like one baby . . .

The one person who wasn't convinced that it was one baby was my amazing—and holy cow, pretty psychic—maternal grandmother.

She was sure that it was twins, and informed the doctor on multiple occasions. She even bought a statue of twins on a trip to Israel and came home and gave it to my mom. At this point my mom's obstetrician thought my grandmother was a total quack.

The doctor couldn't even look her in the eye after he pulled me out by my toes, a bit stunned that I wasn't the placenta he was expecting. My sister was about four pounds, and I was just over two pounds, so when they told my mom that there may be a third, she asked to be put to sleep.

My twin sister, Stephanie, had most of our blood in her body, so the neonatal team got busy transfusing some to me. My dad describes our birth as completely traumatic, especially because so tiny and at five weeks early, he said I looked like a chicken that needed to be plucked. I don't think I was very cute.

My parents tell me that I was a fighter. During my six-week stay in the neonatal unit I received tons of love, thanks to my extremely devoted grandparents and parents. My paternal grandmother never missed a day of visiting me.

I am extremely lucky that I had no long-term issues, and I grew to be a really healthy kid. I've just always been on the small side. Steph is two inches taller than my five-foot-one frame. It must be all the blood she hoarded, but I try not to hold it against her!

I have been lucky enough to not have to worry about my weight for most of my life, but as I began to approach forty, things started to change for me. It used to be that if I put on a pound or two I could just eat really healthy for two days and it would come off. Now, not so much.

I've always had a pair of jeans that were a bit tight in the waist so they looked good in the legs, and I call them my "going out" jeans. Do you have them, too? I am okay with them feeling snug in the waist because I convince myself that I'll eat less when I wear them,

which usually doesn't happen and I just come home with a stomach ache and indentations in my belly. But I digress . . .

When my workout clothes with elastic waistbands began to feel uncomfortable, I knew I had a bigger issue than I ever had before, and it totally freaked me out. I began to reach out to professionals and other people in my life for advice and frankly to commiserate. Some of these conversations made me feel better, while others left me feeling depressed. Like the one I had with my gynecologist.

At one recent visit I saw a number on the scale that I hadn't seen since my pregnancy weigh-ins, and I was not happy. He told me very matter-of-factly that it was a matter of calories in and calories out; now that I was getting older (older!), I didn't need quite so many calories in because my metabolism was slowing down. That was *not* my favorite conversation.

Looking for a medical opinion that I liked better, I visited my primary care physician; I was convinced my hypothyroidism medicine may need to be adjusted. Sadly, I didn't find what I was looking for there either. Unfortunately, even though I had gained weight and felt a bit more tired than usual, my numbers weren't as off as I had been praying they were. That would have been a reasonable explanation that I could have run with. So with a minor adjustment in my medication I moved on to a more holistic approach.

My trainer gave me great advice. She told me to make one small change, for example changing my exercise to shock my body, or making one small change food-wise. I liked her philosophy because it falls right in line with my self-care philosophy in general. Small tweaks and changes can lead to big results.

I had been complacent about exercise for the prior few months, so I recommitted to doing something every day for thirty minutes, even if it was just a walk. I also went back to my in/out rule with

stricter standards. I eat really healthy at home, and splurge on occasion when I am out. I find that if I splurge at home too, then the
splurges become a daily occurrence rather than a special treat.

I also began working with an amazing nutritionist who was able
to help me understand more of what my body needed and was missing. I liked her philosophy as well about staying ahead of cravings,
just like I advocate staying ahead of screaming at our kids by being
mindful and aware of our emotions.

I gained a ton of awareness about what I was eating and how
often I should eat. I tended to graze all day, and she made sure I was
waiting two or three hours between meals and snacks, which was a
big change for me. I did great when I was following her plan, but I
found that I ebbed and flowed in terms of consistency.

Mark thought I was crazy and told me that I looked great. He
actually said that I looked the same as always, which was a total lie,
but it came from a good place. He loves me more than anyone in this
world, and he even thinks I look good without under-eye concealer,
so obviously he is blinded by love.

It seemed that the few good friends whom I confided in about
my struggle, and how it was making me feel frustrated, confused,
and a bit sad, were all going through the same things. Our pants were
tight, but it felt good not to be alone.

The consensus among all of us was that the struggle came from
wanting to feel our best on the inside and look our best on the outside, but we didn't want to think about food all the time. None of
us wanted to feel restricted and deprived or to let food rule our lives.

I decided to give up ever dieting again and to fully embrace
mindful eating. It was time to recommit to the mindful eating strategies that I was so good at teaching others but had thrown by the
wayside for myself.

Of all my self-care practices, mindful eating by far is the hardest one for me. Actually, it's pretty much the only thing for me that feels really difficult in terms of bettering my health and wellbeing. No matter how much I practice, it is something I have to focus on day in and day out.

I thought that my ten-day silent retreat would be the perfect place to hone my skills. As I was preparing to go, I thought about the fact that I was going to have thirty meals with no talking and no distractions. This was the perfect opportunity to up my mindful eating game.

While I was on the retreat I did amazing. I chewed my food completely. I put my fork down between every bite. I didn't feel the normal pressure to finish every bite on my plate. I was a mindful eating rockstar!

I am ashamed to say that sadly it didn't last. I came home and fell into my old habits until I had literally had enough. That, and my various doctor visits and venting to friends finally gave me the push I needed. Even though my weight gain wasn't obvious to anyone who saw me with clothes on, I just didn't feel like myself.

I have used the following strategies on and off through the years, but now that I am using them religiously I am feeling better in my clothes, and most importantly, I don't feel like I am dieting or watching what I eat constantly.

Mindful eating is not about guilt or deprivation. It's about listening to the signals of your body and allowing them to guide you. These are my best tips for making this a reality in your life:

Do a body scan before you eat

I realize that I hold tension in my body before I begin a meal, and this causes me to eat really fast. When I pause before I eat to take a

few deep breaths and notice where the tension is in my body so I can release it, I eat much slower from the onset of my meal.

Bless your food

I didn't grow up saying grace, but it is a lovely tradition. Our food doesn't just appear on our plates. It takes Mother Nature, farmers, truck drivers, grocery checkout clerks, and someone to cook the food for us to eat. By taking a mindful moment to express gratitude for our meal, we can appreciate it for how it is nourishing our body.

I usually say something that I learned from Gabby Bernstein, like "I love my food, and my food loves me."

The upside is that it is hard to bless junk food, so you also give yourself time to get out of a situation you may not feel 100 percent about! Try blessing chips and cupcakes and see if you still want to eat them.

Do you actually like what you are eating?

Not everything we eat is worth it. I think most moms can relate to my opinion that there are good French fries in this world and bad ones. Every once in a while I happily indulge in a few fries that are crispy, salty, and piping hot. To me they are worth it, and I feel no guilt about enjoying them from time to time.

Then there are fries that are cold, mushy, and tasteless. These are the ones that we mindlessly eat off of our kids' plates and then feel guilty and ashamed. We beat ourselves up and wonder why we can't make better choices.

If I am eating something that I consider a splurge, like a dessert or fries, I take a bite and decide if I truly like it and if it is worth it for me to continue eating. I may eat one cold, mushy fry and say, "No way, totally not worth it." On the other hand, I may taste a bite of

heavenly, decadent cake and decide that savoring a few bites is what I want to do. Then there is no beating myself up involved.

Are you really hungry, or is it something else?

Snacking can be really habitual. Maybe we always have a snack when our kids do, or always at 3:00 p.m. or while watching TV after dinner. Just because we have created this habit, it doesn't mean we can't break it! Working from home means that I am near my kitchen all the time. I realized that I had certain patterns around eating, such as eating to procrastinate, eating when I'm bored, and breaking off a piece of dark chocolate from a bar every single day after lunch.

Paying attention to the signals our body gives us around hunger can help to break these habits. Hunger comes on slowly and builds, whereas cravings come on strong and fast.

I heard a tip from a nutritionist recently that really clicked. She said to use the fruit rule. If you feel hungry and would be willing to have fruit, you are most likely legitimately hungry. However, if the only thing you'd be willing to eat is a bowl of ice cream or cookies, you are having a craving.

I have also come to realize that I occasionally eat when really I am thirsty. Sometimes a cup of tea or a big glass of water is what my body is really craving—I have upped my water consumption to hold my body weight in ounces a day, and now that I am properly hydrated, I don't crave snacks all day long like I used to.

Appreciate what you are eating

I have eaten so quickly that I don't even remember tasting my food. My plate was clear, but I kind of missed the meal.

If you can describe the flavors of your meal and the texture of what you are eating, even in your head, you are most likely eating at a mindful pace.

When we appreciate our food it all seems worth it, even the splurges, because we are truly enjoying them. You may only need a bite or two of something rich or sugary because you were able to savor it instead of getting in every bite while you can.

You don't have to say "no" to foods if you eat them slowly, only when you truly want them, and stop when you feel satisfied instead of stuffed.

Put your fork down between bites

It sounds simple, but when you really become aware of this, you may notice that you are already preparing your next bite of food on your fork before you finish what's in your mouth. This can make you feel rushed and cause you to swallow before you've really had a chance to chew your food well.

Slowing down in this way can also help you realize when you are full. If you are shoveling your food and feeling like you have to clean your entire plate, you may miss your body telling you that it's full, and all of a sudden you are overstuffed.

I recently picked up a super fun tip from Robyn Youkilis, a well-known health coach, that helps me to eat slower as well. I place a tiny Buddha statue next to my plate as a reminder to slow down and enjoy my food. My Buddha is a happy Buddha, and his smile makes me smile as I enjoy my food. Many of my clients have adopted this ritual too.

Prepare

The way I prepare for my week has the biggest effect on how I eat for days on end. For that reason I am going to spend some extra time here.

When I take the time to prepare healthy food for the week on Sunday, I notice a huge difference in how I eat all week long. I call it my "Sunday Prep." I take one hour to cook things like lentils, quinoa, oatmeal, hard-boiled eggs, mason jar salads, and roasted veggies that I can put together in different ways to make healthy meals all week.

For example, quinoa can easily be turned into a filling breakfast bowl with almond milk, fruit, and seeds, or I can make quinoa fried rice for a dinner or as a side dish. Lentils can be paired with scrambled eggs, used as a salad topper, or used as a side with any entree for dinner. The best part for me is that I cook as much as I can on the stove at one time and then only have to wash pots and pans one time!

Here are some examples of what I make on Sunday and how I use them:

Steel Cut Oatmeal	Breakfast bowl with unsweetened almond milk, berries, hemp seeds, flax seeds, almonds, and coconut nectar
Mason Jar Salads	Dressing at the bottom, hard veggies, then protein, then lettuces
Quinoa	breakfast bowls, fried rice, as a side with butter and salt, in mason jar salads

Hard-boiled eggs	As a quick snack, in mason jar salads, as a breakfast side with oatmeal, pack in kids' lunches
Black beans	In breakfast tacos, as a side dish
Bone broth	To sip as a warm beverage, use in a latte, to cook with

Having your fridge stocked with healthy options makes it much easier to make mindful choices. I also notice that the way I start my day has a big effect on the rest of it. If I start the day off with a healthy breakfast and mid-morning snack, I am motivated and inspired to keep eating healthfully all day long.

Visit my website, www.hotmesstomindfulmom.com, and get your free weekly meal plan—all of the recipes can be prepped at one time!

The days of eating sushi standing in line at the grocery checkout or while I push my cart to the car are over. I aim to sit down, chew thoroughly, and actually enjoy my food.

Mindful eating can be a reality in your life. Ditch the diets and the struggle around food, and let your body guide you to food freedom. Food can be medicine, and it can also be poison. The better we eat, the better we feel. The better we feel, the more energy we have, and if you are like me, the more patience I have with everyone around me.

Eating healthy meals throughout the day helps me to stay patient and present. When I go too long without food I get hangry and basically turn into a short-tempered bitch. If you ask my husband, he would very much agree! It feels out of my control, but it isn't. I simply need to stay on top of my hunger and have the right foods on hand.

I enjoy modeling healthy habits for my kids, especially my little one. His sweet tooth is absolutely not his fault. All I wanted during my pregnancy with him was sugared cereal. I would spend half my trip to the store deciding between Cookie Crisp or Golden Grahams like my unborn child's life depended on it.

Our habits around food directly affect our children's. This is another area where they learn more from what we do than what we say. You can tell your kids all day long to eat their veggies, but if your hand is in a bag of Doritos when you do, good luck with that!

It isn't always possible to sit down as a family every single night. In my home, sports schedules often wreak havoc on our family dinners. There are nights we wait until 7:45 or 8:00 p.m. to eat as a family, and there are others where it is a free-for-all. One child is having soup before practice, and the other is having breakfast for dinner when they get home. I simply do the best I can and aim for a few nights during the week that we all eat together.

It is virtually impossible to talk about mindful eating, or eating in general, without mentioning self-compassion. Food can trigger judgment, shame, and guilt, but only if we allow it to.

Once I started eating more mindfully, I began to really savor and enjoy treats and only have them when I really craved one, not because I was bored or procrastinating or I felt sad. To help keep the amount of treats I have in check, I also institute the in/out rule. I eat super-duper healthy in my home, and most of my treats are out of my home, with the exception of really dark chocolate. I can't live without a square every day (at least once). Beyond that, most of my splurges are out.

Treats are to be enjoyed, and if eaten in moderation mindfully, it is perfectly okay to have them. The self-sabotage that ensues after we indulge is way more damaging!

I know there are many ways to celebrate as a family, and they don't all have to involve food, but let's face it, many do, or at least in my house they do. After a special performance or ceremony at school, we often get a fun treat like ice cream to celebrate. I want to partake in these celebrations, and I don't want my kids to always see me refrain. I don't want them to think there is anything wrong with having treats in moderation. We strive for balance in life, and food is no exception. If we eat healthy most of the time, an occasional treat is perfectly okay.

I also aim to lead a healthy example for my children as they grow into adults. Restriction is not a viable long-term plan for me, and it's not what I want my kids to see or think is normal. When they think of our eating habits as a family, I hope that their thoughts looking back revolve around healthy choices, occasional treats, and spending time together enjoying our food.

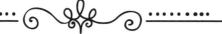

4

Gratitude 2.0

It's not your same old gratitude practice

"Gratitude can transform common days into thanksgivings, turn routine jobs into joy, and change ordinary opportunities into blessings."

—WILLIAM A. WARD

I will never forget when my oldest son was in the school-wide spelling bee. We helped him prepare by testing his knowledge of the words a fair amount (without going crazy). My husband was in charge of the testing process. Our son was definitely prepared after studying every night for a few weeks, and at worst he would not be embarrassed. As I was tucking him in the night before the bee he told me, "Mom, I just want to make it to the top six. If I do that, I will feel really good." So, what do you think happened? I kid you not, he got sixth place. He totally willed it—it was the Law of Attraction, pure and simple. I was completely floored, and after the competition I joked to him that he should have said the only way he would have been happy was if he won!

The Law of Attraction in its simplest form states that we attract whatever we think about, good or bad. I have played around with this concept over the past few years, and I am a firm believer, especially since that spelling bee. I certainly give credence to the fact that our thoughts become our reality, and we have the ability to change our energy with our thoughts.

You know when you just have "one of those days"? You can just tell that your energy is off, and those happen to be the days that every traffic light is red, every salesperson is grumpy and unhelpful, and you spill on your brand new shirt. Once you get into a chaotic loop of negative energy, you call more of that into your day. The good news, though, is that we can take a mindful pause and shift our energy, do something to lift ourselves out of our funk and get into a higher vibration. Maybe it is having a five-minute dance party, taking a walk outside, or watching a funny show—whatever it is, find something that can redirect you back to a present and peaceful place and get your energy feeling high again.

Practicing gratitude is another amazing way to change our energy, raise our vibration, and keep us in a higher energetic realm.

According to many contemporary studies, practicing gratitude brings incredible benefits, such as more positive emotions, better sleep, a stronger immune system, having more compassion for oneself and others, and feeling more satisfied with life in general.

I truly believe that when we live in a vibration of gratitude, the universe gives us more to be grateful for. I am sure you have heard the saying "like attracts like," and in this case I believe it. It's almost like you are telling the Universe exactly what you want more of in your life.

Sometimes I think people feel some sort of pressure, like what they are grateful for must be profound and really major. Some things

are, but there is also nothing wrong with being grateful for a beautiful new lip gloss or shirt. Those things make us feel good, and we can celebrate them. I made someone laugh once because I told them that I bridge the spiritual and material very well. In my book, there is nothing wrong with that!

A client with three little boys once asked me an incredible question: "How do you find gratitude in the chaos?"

As much as we adore our kids, it can feel hard in the midst of runny noses, sibling rivalry, and piles of dishes to feel gratitude in the moment.

Gratitude is extremely important, but there is a time and place where it feels natural. While we are cleaning up throw up or changing a smelly diaper is probably not when we should be expecting ourselves to practice gratitude. There are much better ways to set ourselves up for success! I know you'll love the following concept, and you can think it, write it, or say it out loud in the carpool lane, the shower, or while you are brushing your teeth, if writing in a journal isn't your jam.

There are many simple ways to get your family involved and excited about gratitude as well without feeling like you are nagging them all the time. Here are a few ideas:

- Encourage your kids to think of something they are grateful for in the morning and evening by posting a simple note that says "gratitude" by their toothbrush. Explain that when they see it they should think of something they are grateful for, and then leave them alone about it. I bet they do it and it becomes a habit!

- A colleague of mine once told me that she places dot stickers from an office supply company in random places around her

house. Think next to the salt in the pantry and next to your face cream in the bathroom. Every time you see a dot, you think of something you are grateful for. This too becomes a habit, no nagging involved!

I learned a technique from Mary Knebel, an amazing coach that I worked with to clear some blocks around money that were still impeding my success. The incredible technique is called "Gratitude in Advance." This concept took my gratitude practice to a whole new level. Not only do I thank the Universe for what I have, but I thank it for what is coming, like it is a sure thing. I am basically giving clear-cut directions to the Universe about what I want to happen in my life, and I am saying thank you in advance because obviously it is coming once I take inspired action and do my part by following through on situations presented to me. A very important element of the process is that I then surrender and trust that it's coming and let go of worrying about the how. It is all about releasing resistance and becoming an energetic match for what I want.

I have actually seen things come to fruition from my gratitude-in-advance list, and it is pretty freaking awesome. I have included things like finding my ideal clients, more speaking engagements, an agent and publisher, inspiration for my book, a great new book to read, the perfect ring for my right hand, and new makeup. Just like gratitude in general, My "GIA" can be for big things and small things, too.

Each day I make a two-part gratitude list in my journal. One part is for things that already have happened, and the other is where I give gratitude in advance.

Energy, as well as our vibrations and thoughts, are really cool topics to me, so I spent some time combing through www.highexistence.com

and came across some interesting information about how your bodies react to our thoughts, both negative and positive.

Basically, it explained that there are thousands upon thousands of receptors on each cell in our body. Each receptor is specific to one peptide, or protein. When we have feelings of anger, sadness, guilt, excitement, happiness, or nervousness, each separate emotion releases its own flurry of neuropeptides. Those peptides surge through the body and connect with those receptors, which change the structure of each cell as a whole. Where this gets interesting is when the cells actually divide. If a cell has been exposed to a certain peptide more than others, the new cell that is produced through its division will have more of the receptor that matches with that specific peptide. Likewise, the cell will also have less receptors for peptides that its mother/sister cell was not exposed to as often.

Thus if you have been bombarding your cells with peptides from a negative attitude, you are literally programming your cells to receive more of those peptides in the future. Even worse, you are lessening the number of receptors of positive-attitude peptides, making yourself inclined towards negativity.

It takes more than a few days of positive thinking to make a significant impact on your long-term attitude patterns. Every cell in your body is replaced every two months. So if you have a history of negative thinking, depression, pessimism, or perpetual frustration, plan on working on yourself for longer than a few days before you see more permanent results.

Now when we hear a quote like this from Buddha it makes so much sense: "Your worst enemy cannot harm you as much as your own unguarded thoughts."

That is some serious incentive for keeping our thoughts positive with things like gratitude!

We make choices in life minute by minute, even second by second. Among the most important is where we put our attention. When we understand that we are in control of it, and that we choose what to focus on moment to moment, we are able to be more present and more joyful.

What we put our attention on gets bigger. If we focus on joy, our life feels joyful. If we focus on negativity, our life seems full of it. We have the opportunity to choose how we feel about our life moment by moment based on what we let become bigger. This is an area that I have begun teaching my kids about as well. I want to empower them to realize that they have the ability to make good things bigger in their lives and to minimize negativity if they choose to. The following concept is a great way to explain how to make this a reality for kids.

We can change our negativity patterns by doing what I call "riding the energy elevator." By using your trigger plan (I'll explain this more later), you can shift your energy in any given moment. We don't have to stay stuck in the low-energy basement. We can ride all the way up to the high-vibe penthouse!

As parents we will make plenty of mistakes. In those times, we can focus on what we did wrong, or we can focus on what we learned to make us better, and even get to the point where we feel grateful for the experiences that were difficult. Those mistakes were part of our journey. If we missed them, we missed an important lesson and opportunity to grow.

5

Growth Comes with Recommitment

You will fall off the mindfulness wagon,
but then you get right back on

When I had my babies, there were varying opinions on how to get them to sleep. I had friends in both camps. Some woke their babies every three hours like clockwork to eat and remain on a predictable schedule. Others repeated the mantra "sleep begets sleep" as their babies snoozed and developed their own sleep patterns.

I was insecure and unsure of myself as a new mom, so I remember trying it all! I most likely would have been more successful if I had just followed my gut and done what felt right from the get-go. I probably confused my poor babies!

I imagine if I were doing it again today, having a newborn as the new and improved me—the self-care practicing, more laid-back version of Ali—I would probably fall into the "sleep begets sleep" camp.

I have joked that even though we aren't having any more kids I would love the opportunity to have a newborn as the most present version of myself. I'd let go of a lot of the bullshit, forget about what I was "supposed" to do, listen to my intuition, and let myself simply enjoy the baby phase more. The first time around I was so concerned about doing everything "right" and with keeping up with what everyone else's baby was doing compared to mine. Were we on track? Were we ahead? I was trying so hard to do it perfectly that I forgot to just enjoy the fleeting moments. I mean, of course I cooed and I snuggled and I breathed in that baby smell, and talked to my babies incessantly, but I still paid too much attention to what was going on around us. If I were doing it again, I don't think I would notice half as much.

When I compare how I dealt with insecurities about making decisions when my kids were little, like the best way to get them to sleep, versus the confidence I feel in terms of decisions around my own care and how I care for my family now, I see such growth. These types of decisions used to paralyze me, and they felt absolutely huge, like the weight of the world was on my shoulders. If I made the wrong choice every bit of pressure I put on myself would come crashing down upon me.

So many people are scared and overwhelmed at the thought of making changes in their lives, even though those changes would ultimately make them healthier and happier. Our life doesn't have to be turned upside down when we incorporate change because transformation doesn't have to happen all at once; in fact, small changes can yield big results. Not to mention we can try something, and if it doesn't feel good to us, we can change directions. Self-care and caring for our families never involves the weight of the world. Sometimes it is simply trial and error, but the only way to know is to get started.

The first hurdle is simply getting started

I think people feel intimidated by starting a self-care practice because they think that they need to overhaul their entire life in one fell swoop. When talking change, especially one involving self-care, solidifying one new, small habit and making it stick before embracing another habit is the way to go.

Let's say we try to incorporate daily meditation, a new exercise plan, Sunday prep, a gratitude practice, and journaling all at once. My head is spinning just thinking about it! There is no way that plan would lead to success and any long-term gain. It would last all of a few days at most.

However, let's say we give ourselves permission to make one small addition to our routine, like meditation. Let's say we attach our new habit to something that we already do, like waking up. Every day when we wake up we will meditate for five to ten minutes. That's it. Does that sound so hard? We could procrastinate for months and be scared of it, or we could just get going.

Here are a few ideas for other habits that we can incorporate into our lives, one at a time:

- Thinking of something we are grateful for when we brush our teeth in the morning and evening.
- Remembering to simply thank the Universe that we have the chance to live our very best life again when we wake up in the morning.
- Set an intention each day; an alarm on your phone can be a great reminder.
- Take a mindful minute in the afternoon to breathe and regroup.
- Eat meals only when sitting down.

- Chew each bite of food twenty times.
- Move your body for thirty minutes every day. Walking totally counts.
- Connect with a loved one that doesn't live in your home at least once a day by text or phone.

The same goes for starting new habits and routines with our kids. We can't ask them at one time to stick to a system for completing their homework, cleaning their room every day, unloading the dishwasher each day, and packing their own lunch, or they will probably feel really overwhelmed and do a poor job. However, sitting down and talking to kids about one new habit doesn't seem so crazy. Once the first new habit is up and running, we can talk about bringing another into the mix.

Here is a great list of habits and chores for kids:

- Make their bed every day.
- Think of something they are grateful for every time they brush their teeth.
- Meditate for up to one minute per year of life (a.k.a. how old they are).
- Pack their own snack/lunch for school.
- Walk the dog.
- Stay off social media for at least sixty minutes a day. This may feel really hard for them!
- Do a physical activity for at least thirty minutes a day.
- Help prepare dinner.
- Set/clear the table.
- Load/unload the dishwasher.
- Separate laundry into colors and whites, and maybe run a load.

The second hurdle is staying consistent

Nothing works if we jump around constantly, trying a bit of this and a bit of that. We need to let our practices have time to sink in and simmer in our subconscious so that they become a true part of our routine.

Just like sleep begets sleep, healthy changes in your life lead to more healthy changes.

So what happens when we eventually fall off the wagon at some point? Because we totally will.

One of my favorite sayings that I tell all my clients is "Growth comes with recommitment." We will have off days here and there and we will miss a meditation or making our gratitude list, so don't let it shock you. Don't beat yourself up, call yourself a slacker, or convince yourself that you aren't committed. By simply beginning again, and picking up right where you left off, you are telling yourself that this practice matters to you too much to just say "Forget it."

Coming back to a practice that you value is huge. That is major growth. Having the awareness that you may have hit a bump in the road but it didn't throw you totally off course can boost you up right there.

Life happens, and we need to be realistic about our practices and cut ourselves slack where we need to, as long as the majority of the time we are on track.

I heard a great analogy from a fellow teacher that demonstrates this point perfectly. He was talking about meditation in this case, but I think it can go for any healthy habit for the body, mind, or soul. He said, "Meditation is like taking a shower. You can skip one day of showering and be okay, but if you skip and skip you will eventually start to stink."

Our healthy habits fill us up inside, and we need to remember that practicing them is a gift that we give to ourselves, and we certainly can't forget about our *why*. Why was this habit important to us in the first place? How does it make us feel? How is our life better when we are consistent?

We also have a beautiful opportunity to teach our children about commitment and recommitment. This is not a place to shield our children so they think we are perfect, but be role models by admitting that it can feel hard to stay on track with a healthy habit. By doing so, we can lead by example so when they have trouble sticking to a routine, we can honestly say, "I have been there, too, and I know it can feel hard," and they'll actually believe us.

The third hurdle is creating a new normal for ourselves

We will get to the point where our new habit is so ingrained in us that there is no going back. It simply is a part of what we do. There is no one time frame for how long this should take, and it will be different for everyone and each habit that we incorporate into our lives.

I got to the point where meditation became a natural and fluid part of my morning routine fairly quickly, but other habits, like those related to mindful eating, need to be consciously worked on every day. They don't feel natural yet, but I hope that my commitment and recommitment to them pays off!

I have a few clients who use incentives as a way to motivate themselves to stick to new habits, especially around meditation and exercise. Of course the internal rewards like feeling less stressed and having more energy are paramount, but I say that if a treat for five days in a row of meditation gets you out of bed, go for it!

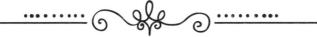

For anyone that wants to use an incentive, I recommend doing it like this, and I will use meditation as an example:

- Meditate every day for five days and reward yourself with something small like a Starbucks stop.
- Meditate every day for ten days and get something a little bigger like a mani or pedi.
- Meditate every day for thirty days and treat yourself to something even bigger like a massage or a new pair of workout leggings.
- Then if you still feel like you need to, you can start the cycle over again.

One final thought that I'd like to leave you with regarding commitment and recommitment is that falling off the wagon at some point is just part of the process. Sometimes we have to struggle so that we can ultimately succeed. Our heart is really in something when we understand how much we want it by coming back to our "why." Our why is the important connection we have to our purpose. It gets us through the fear we face and beyond our inner dialogue of judgement.

If you are struggling with commitment you may need to get quiet and listen to your intuition so you can honor your why. How you want to feel should make your heart skip a beat and your belly do a happy dance. No matter the obstacles, your why is what pushes you through, day in and day out.

6

Make Your Smartphone Your Mindfulness Tool

Don't fight it, use it as an ally

"I like to hang out with people who make me forget to look at my phone."
—UNKNOWN

We all have incredible intentions to be mindful throughout the day, but then life happens and we get distracted and can easily lose our momentum. Emergencies pop up, kids get sick, the sink leaks, the dog needs to go to the vet, and all of a sudden we are back to rushing through the day.

Even though my job is to teach others about mindfulness, I also need daily reminders, and that is where my smartphone comes in. Contrary to what some people think, my life isn't zen 24/7. I always laugh when people say to me, "You must never freak out since you meditate all the time." My kids fight, I forget things on my list at the grocery store, and I procrastinate by skimming my Facebook feed

just like anyone else. Because of these and many other of life's unpredictable moments I know what I need to do to stay sane, and in order to be successful in my mindfulness and self-care practice, I have set up my environment for success. Having tools in place when I need them allows me to recover from life's ups and downs faster and easier. Something may have sent me into a tailspin for days a few years ago, and now maybe it's a few hours, or even just a few minutes.

I don't want to complicate my life any more than it already is between working, being a mom, running a household, needing time for myself, and oh yeah, needing to save some attention for my husband! The reason that using my smartphone as a mindfulness tool feels pretty seamless to me is because I already always have it with me. I am not looking to add any more devices or "things" to my life if I don't have to.

I consider technology a blessing and a curse in my life. I adore how it allows me to connect with others in my business and personal life, and I am always inspired by quotes and posts online. Technology is also one of my biggest time sucks, and I have to be really careful to monitor my time online. But when my phone is used for good, such as helping me to be more mindful, I am glad it is more or less an additional appendage most days.

Here are some ways that I use my phone as a mindfulness tool:

1. I use the reminder feature to flash an affirmation on my screen every hour, such as, "I speak my truth always in all ways" or "Something amazing is going to happen today." These offer me a moment of pause and contemplation even in the midst of a busy day. If an affirmation is especially calling to me, I often use apps like Word Swag or Canva to make a meme and use it as my screensaver.

2. I live and die by my online calendar, and as a working mom I couldn't survive without it. There are days that my schedule can feel overwhelming, but I have programmed mindfulness breaks in to help create space between appointments with clients and chauffeuring my kids. Every single day at 3:00 p.m. an alert goes off on my calendar that says "Gratitude is my Attitude." No matter what I am doing when it goes off, I pause, and after three deep breaths I think of something I am grateful for.

    Getting a second meditation in each day is something that I have really been wanting to do for a long time. I have found that unless I block off the time on my calendar I don't have a fighting chance because there is always something else I could be doing in the afternoon. Now time is set aside each day on my calendar for a short afternoon meditation.

3. The convenience of having my pictures, calendar, e-mail, and even my music all in one place is something that I appreciate on a daily basis. The playlist that gets the most attention on my phone is my "meditation" music. I occasionally do play music when I meditate, or during a class, but I find that this is the music I want to listen to whenever I am alone because it allows me to go within and connect with my soul during quiet times like driving or cooking. Music from Jai-Jadeesh, Snatam Kaur, and Deva Premal are among my absolute favorites.

4. I enjoy journaling but don't always have my journal on me when inspiration strikes and I want to record an important thought. The Notes app on my phone is an excellent stand-in when needed.

5. My smartphone allows me to use mindfulness apps with the touch of my finger, and I am truly grateful for them daily,

especially Insight Timer and The Mindfulness App, which I use to time all my meditations. Using a timer for meditation is essential for a few reasons. The first is that you want to finish each meditation you start, and by timing them you simply meditate until you hear the bell. You can literally set it and forget it and not worry about the time at all. Second, you can set an interval time on the apps very easily. It is important to come out of meditation slowly, so you want to give yourself a minute or two at the end of your meditation to enjoy the silence, set an intention for the rest of the day, say a prayer, or maybe practice a minute of gratitude. On the apps you can set a bell to ring to close the meditation, and another to ring a minute later at the end of your interval. Lastly, the apps use soothing sounds as signals, unlike the timer feature on your phone. I don't ever recommend using that. You spend time in meditation settling your nervous system, and the timer on your phone will scare the living daylights out of you when it rings! These apps also provide the opportunity to listen to a guided meditation, should the mood strike.

7

Ditch Perfectionism and Comparison

They are truly the worst!

"Close your eyes and imagine the best version of you possible. That's who you really are. Let go of any part of you that doesn't believe it."

—C. ASSAAD

Have you ever gotten a stomach ache from Facebook? I have and it ain't pretty for two reasons:

1. I physically feel like crap because tummy aches are never fun. Unless I ask for one, like I do when my kids have a stomach bug. One sip from their glass may (hopefully) kickstart the shedding of a pound or two . . . Have you really never done that?

2. I realize that I am actually having a physical reaction to something that someone else did or said, and I am aware enough to know that means I have unresolved issues around said "something." This means I have some internal work to do.

I am far from crafty, and my kids think that we are making homemade cookies when we add an egg and oil to what comes out of a package. My business is thriving, but I don't make a million dollars while I travel the world. I prioritize my meditation in the morning so my kids' pancakes are microwaved. I know this makes my mother secretly cringe, but she bites her tongue. Trust me, she's had practice.

When my kids were little they were completely cracked-out addicted to the boxed Horizon vanilla milks. I would buy cases at Costco—in fact, that is the only reason I joined. They had one upon waking and one after dinner, and yes, I know that they had something like twenty-nine grams of sugar in each one. As if I didn't worry about the sugar intake enough, my family gave me such hell about them. Since I had to travel 1,500 miles for visits, my family had to stock up on the milks when we were coming to town, and they had better have done the math correctly and multiplied out four per day or I was screwed. During this phase hardly a trip ensued without my family asking me if I knew how much sugar was in them. These stupid milks caused one of the only fights I have ever had with my twin sister.

I can't even remember the finer details, but I remember the actual fight. She said something nasty about the milks and my choices as a mom, so out of defensiveness I retaliated and said something about her parenting which was equally as obnoxious, and next thing we were screaming at each other. Ridiculous! After that I had to have a little chat with whichever family member was hosting me, asking them to please refrain from commenting about "the milks."

Just like every other passing phase, the Katz family graduated from "the milks," but it was my first experience as a parent that led me to feel like I was screwing things up while simultaneously having to defend myself.

I am sure if it wasn't the milks it would have been something else, but in this case I was compared to the mom serving her kids organic skim, while my kids were basically drinking wet sugar morning and night.

There are three types of business in the world. My business, your business, and God's business. Simply put, comparison happens when we veer out of our business.

We all do things differently. Our success as parents isn't tied to how many nights a week we order dinner, or if our kids watch TV during the week. There is no right or wrong, only what works for you. When I think about my success as a parent, I am more apt to consider my kids' manners, their resilience, and if they are nice boys. I always said that I wanted the kids that would sit with someone who was alone at lunch. Some days I think I have those kids, and some days the jury is still out. I may not have the Martha Stewart gene, but I love to snuggle, play games, and I look my kids in the eye every single day and tell them I love them. When I started working and had to calibrate a work/family life balance, I certainly forgot a few things here and there, but hey, it contributed to their resiliency.

As parents we all make different choices, and someone else's choices only seem wrong if we are in their business. I have learned the hard way to just stay in my own. I have given opinions without being asked—a definite no-no—and judged what others were doing, which both stemmed from my own insecurity.

I felt the need to prove that I knew what I was doing because I had all the answers, and now I can see that I was really judging myself. Once I let go of that, and realized that I was enough as a mom, I let go of needing to prove anything.

I began to feel more of a sense of camaraderie with other moms, and less competition. Once I relaxed, my intuition kicked in, and I

felt more confident in my choices and decisions. I began to see what can happen when moms come together to support each other.

When you hear the term "soccer mom," what do you think of? Minivans, Lululemon, and folding chairs? I think of generosity and kindness.

I actually had a mom from my son's soccer team offer to pick him up at a birthday party that her son wasn't going to, and take him to a soccer game so that I didn't miss my other son's championship baseball game. This wasn't even a super close friend, this was simply a mom going out of her way to help me out. What if moms were there for each other like that all the time?

What if we were able to come together to really celebrate each other's wins? I notice that people have a much easier time talking about how they screwed up as a mom, or how their kids failed at something, than about the good stuff that happens. When did celebrating automatically turn into bragging?

A few years ago I wanted to share something really cool that my son did with a friend. I was excited, and I wanted to kvell a bit. I remember saying to her, "Can I brag for a sec?" and then I realized what a negative connotation that sentence had. When we hear the word "brag" we do an internal eye roll. We automatically feel less than the person talking, and our insecurities emerge. So I changed my language.

The next time I wanted to share something positive about one of my kids I asked a friend, "Can I celebrate something with you?" I saw them immediately perk up and get excited to hear what I had to say. Some people may consider bragging and celebrating to be similar, but I feel that they have very different energies and intentions. Bragging is more about being superior, which makes someone else feel less than. Celebrating is more about sharing good news, connecting, and inviting someone into your life.

I'd love to see a shift for more moms so that they feel comfortable sharing the good and bad. People often feel so much more comfortable commiserating about the negatives going on in their lives. It is certainly important to gather support in times of trouble or heartache, but I want to be there for my friends during the good times, too, not just the hard ones. I want to see my friends be happy and excited about what is going on in their lives, and with their children, and I want to celebrate with them.

I don't want my friends to save all the celebrations for the grandparents. I want in, too!

When I was training to get my meditation teacher training certification, we learned about *mudita*, or sympathetic joy. This is simply when we are happy for other people. It is the opposite of envy, and this is something that I practice and practice. Sometimes it feels really easy and effortless. Other times I may notice bits of jealousy arise when I hear about someone's vacation, or their business exploding, but I also understand that if it is possible for them, it is possible for me, too, and I am calmed pretty quickly. When jealousy arises, it is a beautiful assignment and opportunity to examine my own insecurities and establish them as areas for growth. The happier I become with myself, the happier I become with my life in every way. I understand that I am in the right place, at the right time, doing exactly what I need to in order to grow into the best version of me possible.

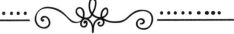

8

Batching

Get more done, better

"We are what we repeatedly do. Excellence therefore is not an act but a habit."
—ARISTOTLE

I live and die by my calendar, and I am not exaggerating even a tiny bit. I probably check it like twenty times a day on average. Not sure what that says about my short-term memory, but moving on.

I've always been a planner and an action taker. All of my bosses and even my husband say the same thing about me: be careful what you ask me to do because it will be done before you have a chance to change your mind!

For years I kept a paper calendar, but after pleading and prodding from a good friend who swore that an online calendar would change my life, I made the switch. Honestly, she was so right, and I wish I'd done it sooner and forgone my terrible system of setting up playdates. I would see someone at school, and they would ask me for a playdate with one of my kids. I would tell them that I didn't have

my calendar on me, but I would e-mail myself to check my calendar when I got home. Then I'd have to check my e-mail to even remember they asked me, then check my calendar and e-mail or call them back. God forbid we had to reschedule and the entire process would start over. Once I switched to an online calendar I could look my schedule up in the hallway of school and enter that playdate right in. So much easier.

I use my calendar to schedule time with clients, but also for things like meal planning, scheduling workouts, planning date nights with my husband or girls' nights with my friends, keeping track of my kids' sports and activities, setting time aside to write or work on projects, and figuring out how to fit in errands between everything else.

What I have found is that batching, which is scheduling chunks of time to get things of a similar nature done, works best for me. I mentioned this in the Sunday Prep chapter in terms of cooking, but I also batch with my calendar in terms of projects and errands.

On Sunday I plan all of my exercise times for the week. If I don't plan them in advance it's easy for exercise to get pushed aside for work, and I can't let that happen and stay sane (or fit in my jeans). Planning ahead also allows me to plan for different types of activities like running, yoga, weights, and walking with friends, which is my favorite social activity. Nothing beats getting in a workout and chit-chat time with a friend, especially outside.

I also make a new list of to-dos for the week. It has two columns: one for work tasks, and the other for personal. Then time gets scheduled on my calendar to make it all happen! I don't do individual errands any more if I can help it either. I will let a few accumulate in the same area of town and run them all at once. Doing so means that I am not running errands every day, and I make much better use of

my time. Once or twice a week I will take care of the personal side of my list, which includes setting aside time on my calendar each week to make household phone calls, order things online, make doctor's and dentist's appointments, and the like.

Work tasks also get batched. I block out times for writing multiple blog posts and newsletters because I find that when I get in the groove and mindset I can get them done more efficiently. I try to see clients on certain days of the week and do work tasks and writing on others. I don't love bouncing from one to the other if I can help it.

Once I have my clients scheduled in, I look at my month as a whole and then plan lunches with friends and bigger household projects, as well as one-on-one dates with my kids. I do my very best to leave Fridays free to batch self-care items like haircuts and color, mani/pedis, and other personal items.

More about the projects

A dear friend, the kind that you talk about the minutiae of life with, told me that she loved how I planned projects ahead on my calendar. She told me that she will never ever forget that she once saw on my calendar, two months in advance, that I had planned to change out all the hangers in my closet on a certain date. I saw an open chunk of time and planned for it so that I wouldn't forget to do it. I do that with tons of big-ticket items such as packing my kids for camp and organizing areas of my house. I need to save the space on my calendar so that those bigger projects don't stress me out because I know I have created time to accomplish them. It may sound anal or insane, but I plan some projects literally months in advance.

It's not just dates and times that I write down, either. When my first son was born, I told someone that I really hope he is super

smart, because I think he took a ton of my brain cells! As soon as I became a mom I started having to write *everything* down.

I always have a huge list going, and if it isn't on the list, it most likely isn't getting done. I have told my husband this countless times. "Don't tell me what you need at the store, *write it down!*" I review my list in the morning and evening, and items get added to the list as I think of them during the day because I e-mail myself constantly. I typically get the most e-mails a day from myself!

I am sure there are many of you that can relate and do the exact same thing, and there are others that think this is way over the top. If you still have a great short-term memory, I am jealous.

All kidding aside, I do really notice that I can be more present during the day once I jot an item down on my list, or journal in the morning. Trust me, I wouldn't add anything else to my routine if I didn't find it absolutely helpful and enjoyable.

The best part is, there are at least a hundred different ways to do this, and they all work. Some people like paper and pencil lists, like me, and others like to keep them electronically. I have a number of friends that swear by the app Evernote, but I am kind of addicted to my legal pad and pen. Find what system works for you and let it all out.

It's amazing because even as list-oriented and planning-obsessed as I am, I have actually chilled out in the past few years. In the past, if I didn't get into bed with every single thing crossed off my list, I would be a stressed-out mess. These days, since I batch and plan more, I know I have time set aside to complete tasks and errands, so I feel more relaxed. And I don't let my to-do list rob me of being present when doing other things like connecting with my family or seeing clients. It's easier for me to relax and truly enjoy what I am doing in the moment when I know that I am organized. I have also chilled out in other ways, too.

I grew up being a total neat freak, but I have relaxed and begun batching my cleaning and organizing around the house as well, especially on the weekends. I used to walk around all day picking up, straightening, and washing every single glass as it was used. I swear, there were days that I never sat down or enjoyed my loved ones because I would just walk in circles around my house making sure that everything was neat. It annoyed me and made me jealous that my husband would be relaxing and hanging with the kids while I felt like an indentured servant. But then it hit me that I had a choice.

I could spend all weekend making sure my house was in perfect order, or I could ease up a bit and relax. I never let things get completely out of control, but I have released the need to impress my babysitters, and things don't always look perfect at the Katz casa on the weekends. I have actually begun to name it "Sunday House." You can sometimes find a few dishes in the sink, blankets unfolded on the couch, and a pile of shoes tossed onto the mudroom floor. The difference is now I am not uptight all weekend, and I have enlisted help to clean everything up.

Before we all head up to bed on Sunday evening, we do a sweep of the downstairs as a family. I usually prefer to straighten the kitchen, and then I assign out jobs to the kids and Mark. Neatness is not one of Mark's many incredible gifts. Mess doesn't bother him, and cleaning downstairs would not happen instinctively, so he gets a job, too. Someone folds the blankets on the couch and puts the pillows back in place nicely, someone organizes all the shoes in the mudroom and someone takes any socks that found their way to the stairs up to the laundry room. We all pitch in to be sure that when we come downstairs on Monday morning the house looks ready for a calm and productive week ahead. I've named this activity our "Sunday Sweep."

I've actually had to become more mindful of enlisting the kids' help and giving them more responsibility around the house. It always seemed easier to just do everything myself, but I realized I was not doing them, their future college roommates, or their one-day life partners any favors!

Of course we started with simple, age-appropriate things like making their beds and clearing their plates. Then we graduated to plates going into the dishwasher, getting fresh water for the dogs, and taking out trash and recycling.

As a serial planner and self-proclaimed "calendar addict," I knew there was more my kids had to understand about organization, and I wanted them to have the tools and executive functioning skills to organize their time and their lives, not just their surroundings.

I gave them each a whiteboard in my office to keep track of their activities, tests, and assignments. They wrote each day of the week and then what was due school-wise and if they had a sport or activity that day. We looked at it together on Monday and planned out a homework and study schedule for the week based on what they had written. For example, if they had a test on Thursday, but there was baseball Wednesday night, they had better start studying for that test on Monday or Tuesday. It is also a great place to make lists of what needs to be taken to each activity, hot lunch schedules, and any other helpful notes.

If your kids need help with planning and organization, I highly recommend this method. I have suggested it to a few clients whose kids have really taken to it. In the beginning you may need to be more involved in the whiteboard process, but eventually school-age kids and older will get the hang of the planning process and be able to handle it on their own. It gives them a sense of responsibility, autonomy, and skills that will last a lifetime.

As moms it is usually easier to do things ourselves, but we aren't helping our kids in the long run. I fight that internal battle all the time! Taking the time to teach these skills now will make life so much easier for our kids in the future. We have the opportunity, and I think the obligation, to empower our kids so that they have a sense of accomplishment and confidence. What a gift for them.

9

How and Why to Have a Mini Silent Retreat at Home

You deserve it!

"In the end . . . I am the only one who can give my children a happy mother who loves life."

—JANENE WOLSEY BAADSGAARD

I don't know about you, but there are days I feel like my self-care is sandwiched between work, making lunches, school projects, homework, grocery shopping, making dinner, doing dishes, and carpool.

Even though I rise before the rest of my household to get in my formal seated meditation, journaling, and gratitude practice, self-care is about way more than that. I like my days to be full of it! For me, self-care includes things like:

- Mindful and healthy eating.

- Exercise, which is good for my body and mind.
- Beautifying with mani/pedis, facials, and haircuts because they make me feel pampered and relaxed.
- Social time with friends over a tea or a walk.
- Time for hobbies like reading and (let's be honest) Netflix.
- Mindful Moments during the day where I can pause and simply breathe and re-center.

This stuff doesn't just happen, and must be scheduled just like a work commitment or activity for my kids. That's right . . . I tell clients to schedule their self-care like it were an appointment for their kids, because we would never cancel those!

The one exception to that is Mindful Moments because I create those all day long, as often as I can. I use typical wasted time like standing in line at the store or waiting in line at the ATM to breathe, calm my nervous system, and think of something I am grateful for. I also give myself a mindful moment as I transition from one activity to the next, such as before seeing a client, before I head out to run errands, or while I'm in the car on the way to get the kids and put my mom hat on.

We must be realistic in terms of what types of self-care we can fit into our day and what feels like a good balance for us so as to not start feeling guilty, fretting, or getting stressed out about our self-care. That seems pretty unproductive and goes against everything we are trying to accomplish. We are trying to make our days better, not harder! Some days are simply better than others. That's why every once in a while I suggest giving yourself a self-care boost where you're not rushed and you aren't squeezing it in. I'm talking about a mini silent retreat.

An at-home mini silent retreat isn't fancy and doesn't cost a dime, but it will do wonders for your sense of inner peace. This is a

few hours (approximately three) that are all yours. Nobody calling your name or asking you for anything. This is just for you.

I remember once when my kids were smaller, my husband asked me, "How many times a day do you think you hear the word 'Mom?'" I replied something like, "Too many to count, in fact I don't think some of them register." When they stop registering, it is a sign that you need to go within and have some quiet time *alone.*

I also know it is time for a mini retreat when I feel like my spiritual practice has plateaued a bit, or I feel disconnected and not as present. Even as a spiritual teacher this has happened to me from time to time, and I know it simply means I have been going through the motions a bit, and I need more time to really connect and be still and quiet.

Maybe a personal day from work is what it takes to make this happen, or if you are a stay-at-home mom you can block off a morning or afternoon. Another option is to take one day on the weekend and divide it up with your partner. You each get three hours to yourself.

Here is a sample schedule of a mini silent retreat from 11:00 a.m. to 2:00 p.m.:

11:00–11:30 a.m.	Meditation
11:30–12:15 p.m.	Mindfully prepare and eat lunch
12:15–12:45 p.m.	Take a slow, mindful walk outside using all your senses
12:45- 1:15 p.m.	Meditate
1:15–1:30 p.m.	Journal and do a bit of spiritual reading
1:30- 2:00 p.m.	Gratitude or Loving Kindness Meditation sounds like complete heaven to me!

Remember, better *you* = better *mom*. The better you care for yourself, the better you can care for everyone you love. Self-care is never selfish. In fact, it makes you a better wife, mom, employee or employer, volunteer, friend, daughter, sister, and everything in between. It's like what those brilliant flight attendants say on every airplane, "Be sure to put your own oxygen mask on before those that you are caring for."

Give yourself the gift of a few hours instead of rushing through your self-care every once in awhile. How often you commit to this extended practice is up to you, but I encourage you to block time off on your calendar, whether it is once a month, once a quarter, or once a year. Really allow yourself to feel recharged and re-energized before you feel burnout as a mom. You deserve it.

10

Push Less, Flow More

You gotta learn to ride the waves

"When little people are overwhelmed by big emotions, it's our job to share our calm, not join the chaos."

—L.R. KNOST

I had an experience that gave me a lot of insight into how I am currently dealing with stress. I am pretty excited because I saw a lot of progress in the right direction here, so instead of you only learning from my mistakes, I actually get to share something I did right. Whoo-hoo!

My kids were home from school on vacation, doing exactly what most kids do on lazy mornings free from their routine. They were watching TV . . . no real surprise there!

This happened to be a morning that I had a brand-new coaching client coming for her first session. I typically schedule all my clients when my kids are in school, but on days off they are used to getting cozy on my bed and either reading for a few minutes like I suggest before they put the TV on, or slyly bypassing my instructions and

simply putting the TV on from the get-go. Either way, they are super good sports, and I am not complaining. Sometimes a working mom's gotta do what she's gotta do.

We often have a weird issue with our TV; the remote control is beyond annoying, and no amount of tech guys coming to troubleshoot can fix it. So five minutes before my brand-new client was scheduled to walk through my front door, the television in my downstairs family room wouldn't turn off. And for some reason it was on much louder than normal. "Blaring" is the best adjective I can think of. Why, of all days, did it have to happen then?

In one single moment I felt my body tense and my breath shorten, and I immediately thought, "Nope! Not this time."

I learned a cool concept in a business coaching group program that I participate in that taught about three ways people live, and it popped into my head in this moment.

It originally comes from a Bruce Lee movie. I am not totally sure how it began circulating in the spiritual business circles that I hang out in, but I am grateful it did. The three ways to live illustrate that the reactions we have in the moment dictate how stressful or fulfilling life can feel.

You can live in rocks

When you live in rocks, everything feels hard, and you are totally inflexible.

You can live in taffy

When you live in taffy, it is like a giant contest of push and pull, filled with tension.

You can live in water

When you live in water, you flow. You are able to bypass things that stand in your way.

So, when faced with the blaring TV and a new client on her way, I decided I was going to flow like water. After all, this woman was a fellow mom, and she had toddlers to boot, so I knew it probably wasn't the first time she would take part in an improvised plan.

My new plan was to have our session outside in my backyard. It was a beautiful day, and I have a pretty nice backyard, so I felt great about my Plan B. My body was relaxed, my breath was normal, and I was really proud that I didn't freak out. I really liked this water thing!

Just in that moment, when I was in the flow and stress-free, my kids tried the remote one more time, and it worked. I am convinced that it only worked because I figured out a way not to stress! I posted something on Instagram one time that fits perfectly with this story, so much so it ultimately became a popular blog post of mine.

"Some days are a total sh*t show, just so you can see how far you have come."

That morning had all the makings of a sh*t show, but I was able to breathe, stay calm, and flow like water around the stress of it. So I feel great about celebrating this with you—that was some pretty cool sh*t!

Kids pay much more attention to what we do than what we say. We can talk to them about staying calm and finding healthy emotional outlets till we are blue in the face. As you go about your day-to-day life, pay attention to how you are handling situations that are hard. Are your kids seeing you curse up a storm, or are they seeing you take a few deep breaths? We set the tone and teach our kids

what is appropriate in life. This is a perfect time to become aware of how you handle your emotions, too. Maybe there is room for a bit more flow.

Another great way to model for our kids is with *start* and *stop* behaviors. The basic gist is this: if we want our kids to do something, we must do it. If we want them to stop doing something, we can't do it either. Some people may disagree and argue that as the adults we should be able to do whatever we want, and our kids need to simply listen to us. In certain situations, of course, but I am going to stand my ground here because this is something I really believe in. Inflexible rules might help create behavioral patterns (at least when you're watching), but modeling good behaviors helps create thought patterns that will allow your child to flow around their own stressful situations. Here are a few examples of what I mean:

- I want my kids to learn when and how to healthily express emotions, so I try to keep my cool in stressful situations and use my trigger plan when I start to feel overwhelmed.
- I don't want my kids to text and drive when they are of age to drive, so I don't do it. (I mean nobody should, but I am extra aware of this.)
- I want my kids to eat well-balanced meals, so I am extra motivated to eat well-balanced meals. We all have occasional treats within moderation.
- I really try to speak in a respectful tone even when I am upset because I want them to learn to do this as well.

The very hardest one for me is yelling from upstairs to down-stairs, and I am still working on this one regularly. I can't stand when my kids yell for me from their rooms or a different floor of the house.

It drives me nuts, and I ask them not to do it. But then I inevitably catch myself calling them to dinner from downstairs when they are upstairs, and I am modeling exactly what I don't want. Rome wasn't built in a day, and now that I have outed myself, I must be more diligent!

Here are more examples of stop and start behaviors:

START	STOP
Positive tone	Whining
Listening	Tantrums
Respect	Ignoring you
Taking a break when needed	Walking away in a huff

By modeling these start behaviors and being sure that our children understand the expectations around them, we can be consistent, loving, and empowering. But most of all, we can maintain our composure as parents and practice what we preach. More to come on this in Mindful Mom Methods!

When practicing and solidifying a new behavior, it's important to remember that it takes time to stick. If you forget now and again, simply be aware and try again. I like to show my kids that everyone messes up and makes mistakes and that we have the opportunity to always choose again. We can't erase what we did, no matter how much we want to, but mistakes ultimately make us better and teach us valuable lessons. Practicing this allows us to be a bit vulnerable with our kids, and I think they need to see this from time to time. It is okay for your kids to hear you say you made a mistake, because doing so gives them permission to do the same.

11

What's a Brain Dump?

Learn to let it all out

"What is it you plan to do with your one wild and precious life?"
—MARY OLIVER

There are times that I feel like my head is swirling with so many thoughts and to-dos. I have work-related items on my mind, lists of household tasks, things to organize for the kids, and grocery lists. Oh yeah, and the overarching goal to stay in the present moment. *Ahhhhh*!

I find that dumping it all out and organizing my thoughts does allow me to stay more present, because once something is on paper it isn't cluttering my thoughts as much. I have a few ways I do this.

This may be a little "woo-woo" for some of you reading, but I have a definite "woo-woo" side that can sound a little "out there" to some people. I am no longer embarrassed to show that side of myself. If you are down with it, great, and if not, try to stay open-minded. I don't try to convert anyone to believe what I believe!

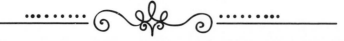

I have had a few readings of my Akashic Records done, which is very cool. Your Akashic Records are the history of your soul: past, present, and future. What I love about these readings is the list of "to dos" that I get from spirit. My friend Shannon, who does my reading, always laughs because she says that my guides and angels know what a "doer" I am and that I like tasks and lists. One idea that came through a reading is that I needed to do more journaling before my meditations. I was going through a period where I felt at a bit of a spiritual plateau. Even though there is no such thing as a bad meditation, my mind was going crazier than usual on a consistent basis, and I just didn't feel as settled into my practice for some reason.

Journaling used to feel like a lot of pressure for me. A big blank page to fill seemed like it would be time-consuming, and what if I didn't have anything to say? I was skeptical, but I always follow through on tasks from spirits, so I sat down with a new journal before my next meditation.

I began doing a brain dump into my journal, and I was floored at how much I had to say. I thought I would write a few sentences, but my hand flew across the page at lightning speed, and all of a sudden I had written three pages. And, I really enjoyed it!

It was surprising how good it felt to be vulnerable with myself and to give myself permission to admit what felt hard and overwhelming as a mom or scary as my business was growing and I was really putting myself out there more. I think it can feel easier at times to resist those feelings and to bury what doesn't feel good, but it never serves us. If we deny our feelings, we can't learn from them, and then the same situations and lessons are presented to us again and again.

From that day on, doing a brain dump before my meditations has become part of my morning ritual. Some days I have a lot to say,

and some days I only write a few sentences, but getting my thoughts out does help clear my head a bit before meditation. That isn't to say thoughts don't still come during meditations, of course they do, but I've resettled into my practice in a way that feels good and comforting.

My journal is also the home for my gratitude and gratitude-in-advance lists. It has become a place where I dream, plan, and sometimes even cry. There are times I am shocked at what actually comes out when I know there is no need to censor anything I write.

12

Work Your Intuition Like a Full-Time Job

That little voice inside your head is there for a reason

"Insanity: doing the same thing over and over and expecting different results."
—ALBERT EINSTEIN

I think I was approximately thirty-five years old before I realized that I even had an intuition since I had never really connected with it before. If I had learned to listen and honor my inner wisdom, I would certainly not have done half of what I did growing up! The more I became aware of the wise little voice inside my head, the more I realized that it gave lots of crystal clear directions, and it was up to me to listen to them. Sometimes I did and sometimes I didn't. I was curious—did I listen more or ignore more? So I began to keep track.

I got a little book, and I started keeping notes on what happened when I heard that smart little voice inside of me. It turns out that it

took me a while to catch on because most of what I wrote were times that I didn't heed the warnings it gave. Here are some examples of when I didn't listen and I should have:

- I had a gut feeling that I should tell my kids that they couldn't play soccer in the house anymore because their kicks were getting too strong, but I got distracted and forgot. A few hours later, my son kicked the ball into my favorite console table, and the leg broke.
- I was getting ready for a party and ignored the feeling I had that I should change into something nicer, and then I got to the party and was completely under-dressed.
- I had a nudge to check my son's backpack for the challah bread that he brought home one Friday, but got distracted. When we got home later that evening, my dog had somehow unzipped his backpack and eaten half of it.
- I knew in my gut that an exercise I was doing at boot camp didn't feel right, but I tried to fight my way through it and ended up throwing out my back.
- I got dressed up early in the day for a birthday lunch, and even though I had a fleeting thought that I should dress casually for carpool and seeing my client and then change afterward, I didn't. I was walking out the door and spilled an entire chai latte down the front of my brand-new blush silk tank top.
- As I was leaving a meeting at school, I had a feeling that I should go check on my son who was coming home in carpool. I didn't because I convinced myself that all was fine, and shortly after I got home I received a call from school that I needed to come back and pick him up because there was a carpool mixup.

- Every single time that I walk out of my house with two poop bags for my dogs because I am too lazy to open the drawer to get a third, even though my intuition tells me to, I end up needing it.
- I was visiting family for a few weeks over the summer and had an inexplicable sinking feeling about my car, so I called my husband and asked him if he had turned it on while I was gone. He hadn't, and I didn't take the logical next step of asking him to turn it on when I thought about it. When I got home the first thing on my agenda was to hit the grocery store, but when I got in my car, the battery was dead.

Unfortunately for me, the list could go on and on, but you get the point. The little voice inside our heads is there for a reason, and that is to guide us. I like to call it our internal GPS system.

I have also noticed that when I lose it with my kids it is usually because something in me is off, typically because I didn't listen to my instincts about a situation. I realized that my internal landscape needed some work, and I had better start heeding the really pulled-together voice of reason in my head.

When I began to listen to my intuition, things began to change, such as:

- I said no to things that I really didn't want to do up front.
- I decided some things felt good in certain friendships and some didn't; for example, I stopped calling people if they never called me back.
- I followed my heart and gut and let my son switch schools a year before his graduation to middle school. My husband and I felt it was one of our best parenting decisions ever.

- I started to slow down in my business and life and take more time to work through ideas.
- I honored my body and what it needed in terms of food and exercise and went gluten-free to help my thyroid condition.
- I began to give myself more time at home that I was craving.
- I lightened my hair, and I love it!
- I gave my kids more time to relax and loosened up our schedule a bit.
- I went on a ten-day silent retreat instead of attending a group program that was hard to say no to, but was what I needed.

I have also learned that in order to hear this reasonable, brilliant voice, I need to slow down, be quiet, and heed the signals of my body and mind. You don't know what you want until you have what you don't want? Listening to your intuition is kind of like that. You don't recognize the signals until you first ignore them, at least in my case. I am now on intimate terms with what gut instincts feel like, and which fleeting thoughts are trying to save me from my own mayhem.

Over time I have come to recognize the strong intuitive connection between the body and mind. We can actually feel the truth, which means we don't have to look so hard. How our intuition speaks to us can vary from person to person. Some people hear a little voice in their head. Others may feel certain feelings in their belly, or their heart beats faster. There is no right or wrong way to connect to your intuition, but you want to start paying attention to what the different signals you feel or notice mean for you.

When we practice with the little things, like taking that challah bread out of the backpack, then hunches and intuitive hits concerning the bigger things like jobs and whether or not to move are easier to spot because we understand our body's signals.

We can help ourselves decrease our stress and worry, and in turn strengthen our faith and trust in the Universe and ourselves when we pay attention to how smart we really are. I don't know about you, but I spent years looking at outside sources for answers and validation, when all along I had just what I needed right inside of me. Trust me, you are smarter than you realize!

Start paying attention to the thoughts you have that come so fast you could miss them. Slow down enough to hear them. Trust your internal compass. Notice what happens in your belly when you make a choice. Do you get a yum or yuck? Understand that these feelings and ideas are there for a reason. Honor them. Take it from me and don't fight it! You will save furniture, clothing, and time if you listen.

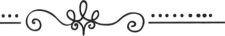

13

The Question That Changed Everything

It's a biggie!

"Successful mothers are not the ones that have never struggled. They are the
ones that never give up despite the struggles."

—SHARON JAYNES

My son totally busted me one day. I was really off, and the best way I can describe it is that I had really messed-up energy while I was driving the boys to school. I felt reactive and on edge. I was snippy and annoyed. I hated the way it felt even in the moment. My son told me, "Mom, I think you need to use some of your own tools." He was right, and I totally got schooled by a ten-year-old.

It is possible to just be "off" sometimes. Even with all the meditation, journaling, and time in nature. We are human beings with hormones and moods, and it just happens. The more I use my self-care tools, and the more ingrained they become in my routine, the more these moods stand out to me because fortunately they happen

much less frequently. But I am not immune to them. And truthfully, because they happen less and less, they really stand out and feel uncomfortable. To me *and* my family.

Once I have become aware of my occasional mood and forgive myself for being human, I can begin working toward reorganizing my energy.

One way that I reorganize my energy is by asking myself this big question: "Is this thought or action taking me toward being the best version of myself?"

I have asked myself this question in a variety of situations like:

- When I've had a judgmental thought toward someone.
- When I am making decisions related to growing my business.
- When I am managing my time.
- When I am practicing self-care.
- When I am being hard on myself.
- When I am choosing foods that will nourish me.
- When I realize that I have been spending too much time on social media.

Sometimes the answer is yes, and sometimes it is no, but it is always a meaningful gauge of how I am spending my time and energy.

If the answer is yes, then I am on the right track, and I feel great about the direction I am heading. If the answer is no, I need to change something about my actions or thought process. I give myself the opportunity to not gloss over a feeling that may be uncomfortable, but instead to really investigate what is going on in my internal landscape. This reflection allows me to dig deep and face feelings which occasionally are not easy to face. Let's say for example that I

am judging another person: that obviously is a sign that I have to ask myself some tough questions as to why and how that judgment reflects on how I am feeling about myself in the moment. Where do I need to do some soul-searching? Is there something within me that needs to be worked on?

I have also asked my kids this question when they are grappling with decisions or issues with friends. Even though they are young, this question makes sense to them. Which direction will make them feel proud, secure, and confident?

My goal in bringing this up in conversation with them is to help them start thinking along these lines, checking in with their intuition, and making decisions that take them toward being the best version of themselves. It took me years to figure this out! Hindsight is 20/20, but what mistakes could I have avoided if I had learned to ask myself this question earlier? That may be another book!

14

Meditation for the Real Mom World

You know you wanna try it!

*"I have come to believe that caring for myself is not self indulgent.
It's an act of survival."*

—AUDRE LORDE

I feel strongly that in order to be successful at anything, we have to understand why we are doing it. For example, knowing why we decide to eat healthy and exercise is essential to sticking with any kind of program. Maybe it is because our doctor suggested it will help lower our cholesterol, or we need to lose weight. But we can and should also take this one step further. How will we feel when we do those things? Will we have more energy to play with our kids, or feel stronger and more confident? The *why* is everything.

Focusing on why we want to meditate as parents is our greatest motivating factor to actually do it. There are incredible benefits of meditation that truly touch our body, mind, and spirit. What I love about meditation is that there is something for everyone, especially as parents.

There are many physical benefits of meditation, such as lowering your blood pressure, helping to regulate your sleep and digestive patterns, helping with chronic pain and ADHD, boosting the youth hormone, and more.

There are also tons of emotional and mental benefits such as becoming less reactive and more responsive, having more compassion for yourself and others, being more connected to your inner guidance system, and feeling less stressed.

I don't know about you, but I think these all sound amazing! I always say I can't tell you exactly what will happen for you, but I know whatever it is, you will like it. I've never heard anyone say that they liked themselves better before they began meditating!

I can tell you from the bottom of my heart that many benefits associated with meditation have made a huge difference in my own life as a mom. I always highlight self-compassion and becoming less reactive and more responsive for parents because they are simply huge when it comes to parenting and are some of the biggest changes I have seen in myself.

Another great one for parents is boosting your immune system. I don't know about you, but I don't have time to be sick.

It also leads to an increase in problem solving abilities. Sometimes I feel like I need a second degree in organizational management to tackle our family schedule and where everyone needs to be and how they will get there, so this really helps!

Raising kids can feel pretty chaotic at times, lots of times, and meditation can truly help to increase feelings of calm.

Next, I'd like to get into the three ways that meditation trains your attention.

Learn to focus on one thing at a time

The first is that it trains your brain to focus on one thing at a time. In this day and age, this is so important. How many times have you been with someone, and in the middle of your conversation they start scrolling through their phone? It doesn't feel very good! We want to train ourselves to really be in the moment so we don't do that to other people.

Think of how your relationships would improve if you were really, truly focused on the person you were with and not thinking about your work or to-do list in the back of your mind. Our spouses and partners, and especially our kids, can tell when we are really listening. Have your kids ever asked you if you are really listening when they are talking? Mine have, and it hurt my heart because they were right. I wasn't listening!

There is a huge misconception out there that multitasking is the way to go, but all it means is that we get more done poorly. If we do one thing at a time, we do it better.

Cultivate present moment awareness

Meditation also trains your attention to stay in the present moment. So many of us spend lots of time ruminating about the past or worrying about the future, even though we want the majority of our time to be in the present moment.

Here's a little secret: nothing we can do will change the past. We have to learn the lesson from each experience, incorporate it into our being, and move on. Some of these experiences and lessons will feel good and some won't. They aren't all comfortable, but they are all necessary! As I said earlier, we have to let go of the past before it

drags us down. There is something else I once read that always makes me feel better. It was that the Universe doesn't do anything to us, only for us. Instead of wondering why things are happening to me in a "woe is me" way, I remember that there is a bigger plan that I just may not be privy to yet, and sometimes I am being cosmically redirected!

In terms of worrying, I like to remind people that there is a big difference between planning and worrying. As human beings partaking in life as we know it, we must plan. We plan for retirement, we save for our kids to go to college, and we organize trips. However, worrying is a totally different energy, a very chaotic one that takes over our present every chance it gets. Here's the crazy thing: 90 percent of what we worry about doesn't even happen. It is insane when you think about it. Our energy and attention goes into something that has a 90 percent chance of not even taking place.

When we find ourselves in a place of future tripping, or upset about something that happened long ago, we need to get ourselves back to the present moment. That is one reason that we practice meditation. In meditation we are focusing on the here and now.

Learn to focus inward

The last amazing way that meditation trains your attention is that it helps you to focus your attention inward. This is especially beneficial for all you moms who usually consider yourself last on your list of priorities.

We cannot fill someone else's cup from an empty one. We must take the time each day to fill our own cup, and meditation allows us to do that. We get to spend a few quiet, peaceful minutes a day refueling and re-energizing ourselves.

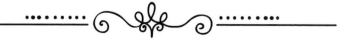

There are five essentials of meditation that I teach, and I love them because they make meditation feel really relatable and comfortable.

The first essential thing to remember is that it's okay to have thoughts. The average person has a thought about every two seconds, which correlates to thousands of thoughts a day. To think that you are going to sit down and clear every thought from your head during your meditation period is completely unrealistic. Trust me, you will have thoughts, and this is totally normal, even for people who have been meditating for a long time.

The second is don't try too hard—there is nothing to force in meditation. Anything that happens is okay. You can't will a transcendent experience, just like you can't help that some days you will be more fidgety (which is actually your body releasing stress). There is no wrong way to meditate. If you are doing it, you are doing it right! The only thing you need to do is set aside the time each day to meditate and have a safe, comfortable spot for your practice.

The third essential thing to remember is to let go of expectations. Every meditation is different. Some days your meditation will fly by, and others you will be dying for it to end. Start each meditation with a beginner's mind, and experience that session as it is. You are doing something wonderful for your body, mind, and spirit, so trust the process.

The fourth to remember is to be kind to yourself. Have you heard the saying, "If you had a friend that spoke to you the same way that your inner voice spoke to you, you would never want to hang out with that person?" We all need to be kinder to ourselves and treat ourselves with more compassion. If a meditation isn't going as you had hoped, don't beat yourself up. Instead of judging yourself, think of how you are taking the time out of your busy day to care for yourself and make yourself a priority. The kinder we are

to ourselves in meditation, the kinder we become to ourselves as we go about our days, and vice versa. Give yourself the gift of self-love and compassion. It can really change your whole outlook on meditation and life.

The way you think about your meditations is extremely important. If you consider your daily practice a chore, it will feel like one, but if you consider it a gift that you are giving to yourself, it will feel like a gift.

The last essential is to stick with it. Of course my goal for you is to have a daily practice. Whether you meditate for five minutes a day or thirty, you will notice a number of benefits, but sticking with it doesn't just mean consistency. It also means that you need to stick with your meditation for the duration that you commit to. If you set your timer for ten minutes, you need to complete all ten. Don't decide halfway through that your meditation isn't going the way you hoped or that you're bored. Set a realistic time for yourself and finish. If you are new to meditation, it helps to start with a shorter time frame and work your way up. Sticking with your time will translate to other areas of your life. It will help you navigate uncomfortable situations with more stamina and ease.

I'll never forget the spin class I was in a few years ago that I really wanted to leave halfway through. I was just getting ready to try to sneak out under the radar when a thought popped into my head. I asked myself, "If this were a meditation, would you stop?" Of course I answered no, and I stayed and finished the class, and I was so glad I did.

There are a few keys to having a successful practice that I'd love to share, and I think they really make a difference.

The first is willingness. The desire to meditate must come from within. Nobody can meditate for you.

Another key to success is consistency. The benefits of meditation are cumulative. It is better to meditate every day for a shorter time than to meditate for longer twice a week. Remember, we are clearing stress from our bodies every time we meditate. It's kind of like dusting from the inside. We can't let that stress build and build and think we will clear it out every once in a while with a single meditation. We need to keep our bodies clean inside every day, just like bathing for our outside.

Your attitude toward your practice is essential to your success as well. I mentioned this previously, but it is so very important that I am going to tell you again.

If you consider your daily practice a chore, it will feel like one, but if you consider it a gift that you are giving to yourself, it will feel like a gift. I promise this can make or break your practice.

Now that we have thoroughly covered how meditation can help you, it is time to get into the finer details of how exactly you meditate.

When you meditate you always have a focus, such as your breath, the sensations of your body, a mantra, a candle, or the sound of a voice (if you are doing a guided meditation). When you notice your thoughts wandering during meditation, you simply bring your attention back to your focus. Your focus acts as your home base, so you always know where to go when your mind wanders.

In the beginning this could be every few seconds, but the more you meditate the longer you will notice the periods grow in between thoughts.

(If you want to practice with different focuses, sign up for my free five-day guided meditation challenge in the "freebies" section at www.hotmesstomindfulmom.com. Each day you will receive a different guided meditation sent right to your inbox!)

New meditators always ask when the best time to meditate is. I always tell them it is whatever time you will actually do it! In all

seriousness, you have the best chance of making your new meditation habit stick if you meditate at the same time every day in the same place. This is really personal. You need to find what time of day works for you. For many, I'd say most, people, this is very first thing in the morning. Deepak Chopra uses the initials RPM which stand for Rise, Pee, Meditate. Parents often set their alarm for a few minutes before their kids get up so they can get an uninterrupted meditation in. Some parents wait until their kids are dropped off at school, working parents sometimes meditate during their lunch hour at work, and some before going to bed at night. There really are no rules.

And remember, you can try something out to see how it works for you, and if it doesn't feel like a fit, try something else. You can date a meditation time for a bit before you marry it!

Sometimes people don't want to meditate because they think they have to sit in a funky or uncomfortable position to do it, which is not true at all. When I first meditated I sat in the step of my bathtub with a towel under me. I don't know why that appealed to me—I guess it was near the toilet after I did RPM!

You can meditate sitting on a chair or couch with your back supported and your feet flat on the floor (or your feet on a pillow if you are short like me and your feet don't reach the floor). You can sit cross-legged on a chair, cushion, or couch if that is comfortable for you, too.

If you are sitting on the floor, you want something under your bum, like a cushion, yoga block, blanket, or even a towel. It is difficult to maintain good posture sitting flat on the floor; you want your hips to be higher than your knees.

I do not recommend lying down to meditate unless it is before bed and your goal is to fall asleep. This is because we have been conditioned since we were babies to go to sleep when we lie down, so if

you are tired when you are meditating and you are lying down, you will probably fall asleep. This means you need rest, but a nap doesn't count as a meditation!

Your arms should hang comfortably, and your hands can be on your knees or in your lap and can be facing down or up, whatever is comfortable for you. I prefer mine down.

You want to be sitting upright, but not uptight. Your back should be erect, but doesn't have to be like a rod. You can tuck your chin ever so slightly so that the top of your head aligns with the ceiling.

And then you just have to try it!

If you are a list person like me, here are the steps written out for you:

1. Get into a comfortable, upright position, either sitting on a chair, cushion, or against your headboard on your bed.
2. Set your timer.
3. Begin by taking a few nice, long, slow, deep breaths.
4. Do a body scan starting at the top of your head and moving toward your toes. Look for places you are holding stress and breathe into them so they can relax.
5. Settle into your focus, whether it be your breath, your body, or a mantra.
6. When your mind wanders, simply return to your focus. Over and over.
7. Meditate until your timer goes off, and then sit for another minute or two of an integration period. You can sit and just enjoy the stillness, practice a bit of gratitude, set an intention for the day, or say your own silent prayer.

I have had many clients ask me how to talk to their kids about meditation, and how to get their kids to try it, too.

When I started meditating, my kids were about five and seven. They were definitely curious about the times they saw me sitting quietly with my eyes closed. Even though I tried to meditate before they woke up, my kids have always been early risers, so they saw me meditating quite a bit. At first they interrupted me *all* the time to ask me questions that were of no urgency and could totally have waited. I had to train them that if I was meditating they were not to interrupt me unless it was a true emergency like one of them threw up or was bleeding. It was only a few minutes, and they needed to learn that my meditation time was really important to me, and I needed to focus.

I explained to my kids that when I take a few minutes for myself in the morning to sit and breathe, I can be a better mommy all day long. I can be more patient and pay more attention to them. They totally got that and really learned to respect my meditation time.

I also told my kids that they were *always* welcome to join me during my meditation time if they wanted to be near me, they just had to be quiet and respectful. I encouraged them to come sit next to me and just lay down and relax in the quiet space, or to bring a book in and read quietly if they wanted, or to breathe along with me. They were never excluded from my practice, but they were also never forced to participate.

I started teaching my kids some really simple breathing techniques, which I will share momentarily, for when they wanted to meditate, too. One of my absolute favorite memories is when both kids came in my Zen den to meditate, and one sat under a blanket with his knees up, creating a little meditation tent, and the other brought in an enormous stuffed dog and used it to lean on. It was the cutest thing ever, and this sweet, simple memory always brings a smile to my face!

A good goal for kids is to meditate up to one minute per year of their life until twenty years old. So, for example, if your child is eight, they can work up to an eight-minute meditation. I usually start young kids under eight with even just one minute and work up. Start kids over eight with two to three minutes and work up from there. When I taught my son's fifth grade class to meditate, they started with two minutes and added one minute each week. The kids all loved it, and his teacher said it really helped the environment in the classroom.

Here are some really simple ways to get kids to meditate:

- Teach them to belly breathe; they can sit up or lie down (even though I don't recommend adults lie down, kids don't fall asleep as easily as we do!) and they can put their hand, a small stuffed animal, or a crystal on their belly. Tell them to watch their hand, stuffed animal, or crystal move up and down as they breathe.
- Tell them to pretend they are blowing up a balloon in their belly when they inhale, and they are letting all the air out of the balloon as they exhale.
- Match their inhale and exhale; it is really simple for most kids to match their inhale and exhale. Just like you do, have them inhale for a count of three, and exhale for a count of three.
- Give them a simple mantra—my kids like "in, out." On their inhale they silently think "in," and on their exhale they silently think "out."
- Peace Begins With Me—this is a great Peacefinder Practice, which is a way to deal with stress in the moment to regain a feeling of peace. Go to page 14 for more info! (I learned

the concept from my teacher and mentor, Sarah McLean).
Kids *love* it!

My advice is to encourage your kids, but don't force them. With
kids that are a bit older, when you feel that it is age-appropriate based
on their level of maturity, you can explain more of the benefits of
meditation. Young kids should understand that it helps them to con-
centrate better and to feel more relaxed. Kids who are a bit older may
like to understand how it trains their attention and does things like
boost their immune system and makes them more compassionate.

The cool thing is that we are normalizing meditation for our
kids. When they see us do it, they realize that it isn't some weird,
woo-woo thing that only hippies do. When they notice changes in
you, they will really get interested as they witness it working!

Kids can also use one-minute meditations as needed before tests,
before a sporting event, or in a tough social situation. The more they
practice, the more natural it will feel to use these tools in the moment. We can explain to kids that many of these Peacefinder Practices can be done without others around you even knowing. They
can do deep breathing or "peace begins with me" in their head, and
it wouldn't be obvious to anyone else.

Kids need to understand that they can take a moment whenever they need to, no matter what anyone else is doing, to care for
themselves. If they need a moment to breathe before a test or sporting event, they should honor that need. And we don't have to talk
to them like they are toddlers anymore. We can explain that when
their nervous system is calm, they can become more focused and less
anxious.

I have a great visual that I use with kids to explain how meditation and Peacefinder Practices help them as well. I call it a mind jar,

but there are tons of names and they are widely used by meditation and mindfulness teachers who work with kids.

The mind jar is simply a mason jar filled with warm-colored water, glitter, and glitter glue. It acts just like a snow globe does. When you shake it, the glitter goes crazy all over the jar, but when you set it down on a solid surface, the glitter settles down.

I explain to kids that the glitter represents our feelings, thoughts, and emotions. Sometimes they feel really crazy and feel like they are everywhere, just like the glitter when we shake the jar. But when we set the jar down, the glitter settles, just like our mind and body do when we rest it in meditation or a Peacefinder Practice.

The mind jar can also help the kids to meditate when they watch the glitter settle. Remember, when we meditate, we are settling down the nervous system and focusing on one thing at a time. When kids watch the glitter settle they are incredibly focused, and their system settles, too. It is a perfect tool to use with younger kids, especially eight and under.

Another fun, and kind of sneaky, tool is to have your kids partake in a straw race with you. All it takes is a straw and a cotton ball for each of you. You win the race by blowing in the straw to move your cotton ball to the finish line. Kids are having so much fun that they don't realize that they are taking big breaths to settle down their nervous system. This is fun to do down a long hallway, across a table, or the kitchen counter. I bet you'll have a blast, too!

15

Feels Too Big? Break It Up!

Too much to do? You don't have to do it all at once

"The biggest mistake I made as a parent is the one that most of us make. I did not live in the moment enough. This is particularly clear now that the moment is gone, captured only in photographs. I wish I had treasured the doing a little more and the getting it done a little less."

—ANNA QUINDLEN

My morning routine has grown over the years. It started simply as an eight-minute meditation, so I just set my alarm for ten minutes earlier in the morning and I was off and running. This is exactly how I tell all of my clients to start as well.

In time, my practice began to grow and change. My meditations slowly increased in length as I felt ready. This is another thing that I tell my clients. Only they know when they are ready for more. I don't hand out a schedule that tells them when to bump up their time. When their meditations consistently feel like they are flying by, and they aren't ready for their timer to go off, then I encourage them to

add a minute or two. I now meditate for about twenty minutes in the morning, but there is also more to my routine now.

As I said, this took time, but I now grab my journal before I meditate and do my brain dump and gratitude/gratitude-in-advance lists. Then I meditate, which always ends in prayer. After I meditate I usually read a short passage of spiritual reading. My all-time favorite book for this is *Journey to the Heart* by Melody Beattie. I also love a *A Year of Miracles* by Marianne Williamson. I then pull an Angel Card for myself in order to receive additional guidance, or an answer to a question, and I finally close by using my pendulum to protect my energy for the day. Phew! It sounds like a lot when it is all written out together, but it is such a habit now and it really flows for me.

I typically give myself a minimum of forty-five minutes. If I can get downstairs a few minutes early and my dogs are quick about their business in the backyard, I'll happily extend my meditation to thirty minutes. I don't mind getting up early; in fact, I relish the house being quiet during my spiritual practice time. I set my alarm for some time between 5:45 and 6:00 a.m., and I need to be upstairs getting dressed for the day by 6:45 a.m. so I can be downstairs with the boys by seven o'clock—we typically leave the house at 7:30 a.m.

Most people don't have as many "add-ons" as I do, and some have none. It is a meditate-and-go situation, especially in the beginning, and if that feels good forever, then stop there. There is no need to add anything onto your practice unless you feel explicitly called to. It doesn't make you a better meditator or a better person. This is all personal preference. I tend to veer to the "woo-woo" side of things in my personal practice, but I keep my teaching practice very mainstream and straightforward.

I do have a few clients who tend to veer toward a longer spiritual practice full of journaling and prayer, crystals, cards, and other para-

phernalia, so I wanted to touch on this topic for any of you that deal with longer practice periods, or may one day as your practice expands.

Many moms with young children are also not morning people. They don't want to wake up an hour before their kids, and I totally get that. The good news is that you don't have to!

You can break up your routine any way that feels good for you. Here are some simple suggestions to make that happen:

- Choose what time of day you will be meditating and be as consistent as you can.
- Find a time of day that gratitude feels right for you. Maybe it is practicing it with your kids at the dinner table. Maybe you have a note that simply says "gratitude" on your bathroom mirror, and you think of something you are grateful for every time you brush your teeth. Maybe you connect the habit to turning on your car. Every time you turn on your car, you think of one thing you are grateful for.
- Prayer can be done anytime, anywhere! Traffic lights, in line at the grocery store, or while working out . . . you can talk to God, Spirit, the Angels, the Universe, Jesus, or whatever (or whomever) feels good to you any time you want to.
- Keep a one-line-a-day journal next to your bed, and each night write one great thing that happened that day or a lesson you learned.
- If you are into angel or tarot cards, pull one in the afternoon as a little pick-me-up!
- Set an alarm on your phone for one or two times a day that simply says "breathe."

When figuring out what works for you, remember my golden rule: you can always change your mind!

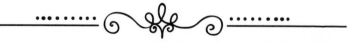

If you don't like how your practice is going, or something doesn't feel right, change it! You don't have to answer to anyone but *you*!

I also want to touch on the fact of how easy it is to get "shiny new object syndrome" when it comes to self-care practices. It happens easily because they all make us feel so good, and once you start learning about self-care, the more you want to do!

My best advice is to go slow. Pick one thing to start with and be consistent so it has a chance to work for you. When that practice becomes a habit, and is really ingrained in your routine, think about adding something else in if you feel called to.

If you jump from meditation to crystals to essential oils to journaling without giving anything a chance to truly work for you, I don't think you will get the results that you are looking for. The rule of thumb is go slow!

That being said, if you try something and truly give it a chance and still don't feel connected to it, maybe it isn't a love connection. Remember, we can (and should) date something before we marry it. Just because your friend is obsessed with crystals doesn't mean you will fall in love with them, too. I mean, you may, and that's great if you do, but different people connect to different practices. Be honest with yourself and what feels good to you.

Keep in mind that different events in your life and different cycles of growth may connect you to different practices. Just like some friendships ebb and flow, your connection to a self-care practice can, too. Just roll with it. You will most likely find something that is a non-negotiable for you, like meditation is for me. I know in my core that this is a lifetime practice for me (okay, I really hope it is for everyone!). I may leave my crystals at home on a vacay, but I will meditate every day while I am gone.

16

Daily Intentions

What do you want to bring into your day?

"Everything that happens in the universe begins with intention. When I decide to buy a birthday present, wiggle my toes, or call a friend, it all starts with intention."

—DEEPAK CHOPRA

My morning prayer is the same every single day of my life, and it goes like this:

"Spirit, Angels, Guides, God, Universe, Archangels, Ascended Masters (I like to cover all my bases . . . sometimes I add specific names as well),

Please be with me today as I strive to be the best version of myself possible. Please help me and guide me as I aim to come from a place of love, gratitude, faith, kindness, acceptance, and patience. Let me find joy in everything I do today. Please help me be a vessel for the right words and the right deeds as I go about my day. Thank you."

I think of my prayer as my intention for the day. It's a hefty one! Intentions don't have to be this all-encompassing, though.

They can consist of something simple like:

- My intention for the day is to meditate.
- My intention for the day is to nourish my body with healthy food.
- My intention for the day is to practice one form of self-care.
- My intention for the day is to speak my truth and stand up for myself.
- My intention for the day is to practice patience with my children.
- My intention for the day is to listen with love.
- My intention for the day is to spend ten minutes outside.
- My intention for the day is to connect with someone I have been meaning to call.
- My intention for the day is to practice gratitude.

Setting an intention is a low-pressure exercise. You don't have to report to anyone what your intention is. A lovely time to set your intention is after your meditation if you practice in the morning, or maybe when you first wake up. Intentions can be written in a journal, spoken out loud, or simply thought.

Intentions can bring so much to your life, especially when you take the actual meaning of intention, which is to aim or plan. You are setting the stage for what you want to see in your day. It can be how you want to show up for yourself, how you want to feel during the day, or something that you want to accomplish. The only thing you need to remember is that intentions are always positive. Like attracts like, just as we've talked about before.

I love this question from *Movement for Modern Life:* "What if you lived today on purpose?" Setting an intention allows us to part-

ner with the Universe to make things happen. We let it be known what our intention is and take inspired action as we go through our day, knowing that the Universe has our back and often takes care of a few details for us along the way. The crazy synchronicities that happen throughout the day which push you in the right direction? Yup, no accident!

Our intention can also help us make better decisions as we go about our day. For example, is eating that double bacon cheeseburger taking us toward our intention of nourishing our body in the best way possible, or would a whole grain and veggie bowl be a better choice? Is letting a friend railroad you into buying something you don't want or need taking you toward speaking your truth and honoring your needs? Probably not. Your intention is another checkpoint to make sure that your internal GPS is on track.

You can bring your kids into your routine as well by letting them know that you set an intention each day, which is kind of like making a wish for what you want to bring into your day, and letting them know that they can join you in your practice.

You can set intentions as a family during breakfast, on the way to school, at the bus stop, or snuggling in bed if you still go in to wake up your kids.

This is a beautiful pause to take as a family during the morning rush of showers, getting dressed, downing coffee, and hurrying the kids through breakfast and out the door. Sharing a mindful moment together can be really bonding and meaningful.

17

Mindful Moments to Start the Day

Even a moment can go a long way

"Our intention creates our reality."
—WAYNE DYER

You know those mornings where the kids are fighting in the car on the way to school, someone gets out crying, and everyone feels terrible? Those are the worst! I do everything in my power to send my kids off for the day feeling centered and ready to tackle the world.

One of my favorite tips for doing this is to practice what I call "morning mindfulness" with my kids. In the car on the way to school we all take three nice, long, deep breaths and think of something we are grateful for. This way I am confident that they are getting out of my car with a calm nervous system and a full heart. One brilliant client of mine shared that she added on setting an intention with her kids to this practice. I have totally borrowed her amazing addition and started doing this with my kids, too.

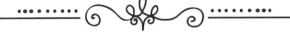

Creating a positive mindset in the morning can help kids deal with social anxiety, nerves before a big game, or worries about a test. Kids can get so anxious and psych themselves up leading up to something that it is going to be so horrible, when in actuality the real experience isn't so bad. Worrying doesn't change having to do it, and since it usually isn't as hard as one thinks it will be in the end, it is a shame to constantly be stealing joy from the present moment. When kids learn to recognize their patterns of worry, they can catch themselves in the act, and now they will have the tools to regroup as they begin a new day.

This can also be done at the breakfast table, walking to the bus, or during a morning snuggle session. Your kids may get into the habit of doing this on their own if they are on the older side, or you can keep it a family affair.

I have a reminder that goes off on my phone every day that says, "My intention for today is . . ." and I take that opportunity to set an intention, but I had never brought my kids into the process.

Our intention for the day should be based on how we want to feel. I often set the intention to feel joy in everything I do. There is no way to mess up intention setting because it is so very personal. We can talk to our kids about what our days would look like if we felt confident, supported, or proud.

Intentions can also help us to choose our thoughts and actions for the day. We begin to understand that we can become an active participant in shaping our reality by putting our awareness on what we want to become bigger in our lives.

Practice setting an intention for yourself every day, and after a few days or a few weeks (you'll know when), introduce the concept to your kids. To start, I would make it more of a conversation, and once they get the hang of it, everyone can set their own daily in-

tention, silently if that feels best. You can ask your kids questions like:

- What good do you want to bring into your day today?
- How do you want to feel at school?
- How can you best love yourself today?

Intentions are different than goals. A goal is to go to the gym five times this week. An intention is to feel healthy and to love your body. Intentions can be what we want to bring into our life, or something that we want to let go of. Intentions are heart-centered and evoke a feeling. Here are a few examples:

Great ones for Mom:
- I intend to use time productively today.
- I will not take things personally.
- I intend to deepen my relationship with _____.
- I intend to release all judgement of myself and others today.

Great ones for the kids:
- My intention is to think only kind words about myself today.
- My intention is to take my time and answer all test questions without rushing.
- My intention is to not feel pressure about how to act around my friends.
- My intention is to take three deep breaths when I feel frustrated.

I have begun incorporating something similar into my meditation practice, and it has become a valued addition to my practice. When I close my eyes and begin taking deep breaths, I think about

what I want to let go of, and how doing so can make space for something I want to bring into my life. For example, "I want to release all
my doubts and judgment about myself today so that I can make the
space for more confidence and authentic connection." It is almost
like a double intention. I am letting go and bringing in. This is simply another way to do it that feels good to me. It came to me when
I was leading a meditation to manifest for a group of women, and it
felt good to all of us. It's another option to try!

18

Turn Your Parenting Challenges into Wins

What can we learn from the tough times?

"Being a mother is learning about strengths you didn't know you had . . . and dealing with fears you didn't know existed."

—LINDA WOOTEN

I start all of my coaching sessions the same way. Before we dive into our work for the day, we always start with wins and challenges. My clients give me their laundry list of great things that happened since we last spoke along with some challenges they faced. Some weeks the wins overtake the conversation, and others the challenges.

One of my favorite parts of this practice is what happens when we talk about the challenges. We talk about the lessons that were learned, how they grew as a person, and what opportunities the situation ultimately brought to their life. By the time we are finished talking about all of this, their challenges look a lot more like wins!

Our challenges are wins because they not only teach us lessons, but they show us where we have room to grow and expand. They aren't always fun, but they are necessary for optimum development.

When I screw up, which is more often than I sometimes like to admit, especially as a mindfulness expert, I am currently much more apt to think about how the experience affects my growth than I am to beat myself up for hours on end, which doesn't help anything.

Beating myself up doesn't change the fact that I messed up, but it does keep me stuck in a place of regret and self-loathing, which is a far cry from growth. It's really either/or. We stay stuck or we allow growth by showing ourselves compassion.

There are times when I say something stupid that I ask myself, "Why can't I just be a shy and quiet girl who doesn't speak much?" But that isn't me. However, I have found more balance between pausing and being more mindful of what I say and blurting out something silly, which is major progress.

When we make mistakes with our parenting, and we will, we need to offer ourselves the same compassion. These situations ultimately make us better parents because we have the opportunity to know what works and where we can improve.

Nobody is perfect, and our kids need to see that so they aren't afraid to make mistakes in life. In fact, when they are young is the perfect time for them to learn from their mistakes. In the grand scheme of life these mistakes will be relatively small (hopefully), and you will be there to talk to them and make sense of a possible solution. We want to arm our kids while they are young with tools like self-compassion, the art of apologizing, how to self-reflect on lessons learned, and how to move past mistakes with ease. I can't even imagine what my life would have been like if I had learned these tools at a young age! Sadly, I have probably spent half my life unnecessarily beating myself up.

There are too many places that I have made mistakes to count, both big and small; in fact, a number are recounted on these pages! One more that I can share, just for good measure, is my all-time personal best. When my husband and I had been dating for about three weeks, I asked him to drive me to the airport when I was going to Israel. I had actually signed up for the trip with an ex-boyfriend, but we broke up beforehand and he backed out. I, craving adventure, decided to go by myself. It was an organized trip, but I didn't know a soul. Anyway, Mark, who was my new boyfriend at the time, got a porter to help me with my bags, and this nice gentleman kindly told me, "Honey, your flight leaves tomorrow." I mean, who the heck shows up to leave on an international trip on the wrong day? At least I was early and not late—could have totally been worse! It has also given my husband a really good story that he loves to share, so, kinda worth it. When my kids heard that story for the first time, their eyes got really wide and they broke out into hysterics. I will gladly take on the role of "mistake maker" for them so they can see how normal and how much a part of life our mistakes are.

I feel able to share them because I have released my screw-ups and I have found gratitude for the chance to learn and move on with more knowledge and grace. This whole book is an example of humanity and truth. It's through our mistakes that we learn the most about ourselves and our children. How can we improve? How do they need us to show up for them? What gifts and passions do we bring to the table? I share my story so other moms feel less alone in their less than finest moments.

But on the flip side, I won't minimize my wins as a parent either. Wins shouldn't be pushed aside; they should be celebrated! There are times that my husband and I look at each other, and without any words spoken, our looks convey our pride in a good decision made.

I'd say a top one so far was when we allowed our kids to attend different summer camps in order to flourish as individuals, convenience be damned.

Parenting consists of good days and challenging days, as well as good moments and tougher ones. I feel empowered to know that moment to moment I have the ability to learn and grow. A mistake in one moment doesn't have to define my next one. It can be onward and upward if I decide so. What will you decide?

Section 2

Mindful Mom Methods

Some people think that the internal work we have to do is the hardest. Maybe they don't have kids! Kinda kidding, and kinda not.

When we do the internal work, it is a choice we personally make because we know our life will be better in the long run. Our kids may not understand that the changes we are making, and in turn asking them to make, will benefit them for the rest of their lives. We want to get through to them and get them on board with our program without hounding them. We want to make mindfulness feel like a seamless part of family life. With time, it becomes the framework for calmer interactions and more loving communication in the home. It feels so good to have tools instead of just yelling all the time!

This section is filled with ideas for ways to set up structures in your home that work for you and your kids. They may not even realize things are "changing," but I bet they will notice that the feeling in the home feels more relaxed. I share simple suggestions for setting

expectations and boundaries in a comfortable and meaningful way, while simultaneously creating an environment in the home filled with love and respect that is mutual between parent and child.

As I mentioned earlier, it isn't our job to be our child's best friend. It is our job to teach them about important life skills and things like our family values, empathy, kindness, unconditional love, commitment, authenticity, and resilience. Because of everything you have learned in the previous chapters, you will feel really prepared to model more mindful behavior. Remember, our kids pay so much more attention to what we do than what we say. That is why the first step was changing our internal landscape and mindset. Now we can bring this wisdom and positivity to our families in a way that sets everyone in the home up for success.

19

Technology Detoxing
Us and the kiddos

"Almost everything will work again if you unplug it for a few minutes . . . including you."
—ANNE LAMOTT

I told my son that I was going to invent a special hearing aid that automatically turned on as soon as a device such as a television, phone, or iPad was in his immediate sphere so he could actually hear me talking to him when he is using technology. I was totally kidding, of course, but only because I am not that techy and I don't know how to go about inventing that. I would actually love a hearing aid like that for my kids—and husband, too, for that matter!

I wrote earlier about how technology can be used to our advantage to make us more mindful, but let's be honest: unless we are mindful about the amount of time we spend using technology, it can also become a major time-suck. Technology isn't going anywhere, so just like eating healthy and having treats, it's all about balance. We

need to give ourselves breaks and do what I call a technology detox every once in awhile.

Have you ever felt an incredible urge to get the adorable picture you just took of your child up on your Facebook page so that you actually stopped what you were enjoying in the moment to make that happen? Me too, but you know what? It totally could have waited. It would have made absolutely no difference if I shared that pic immediately or in a few hours. Instant gratification and instantaneous posting are so ingrained in us these days that we don't even realize that we lose the present moment in the process.

Now that I have a preteen with a phone, I am absolutely amazed at how much time someone can spend on a device (other than reading a Kindle book, which obviously doesn't count). Given occasional free reign, my son can post and watch videos for hours on end—over, and over, and over. My son isn't any different than other teens or preteens on this planet. Most of them are glued to their devices.

According to an article in the *Washington Post*, teens spend an average of seven and a half hours a day consuming media such as television, video games, social media, and music. Teens on average also text sixty times per day. It's a little shocking.

I started to wonder how these habits develop, and it is no surprise once I began looking around. Almost every time I pulled up to a traffic light and glanced over at the car next to me, the driver was on the phone. Nearly every person in line at the grocery store was on the phone. Doctors' waiting rooms, restaurants, and even my gym are filled with people using technology.

I am not immune to this phenomenon. I often read on my iPad and binge watch shows on Netflix. I check my social media business page multiple times a day, and I am writing this book on a computer.

An article on DailyMail.com stated that, "People spend an average of 8 hours 21 minutes sleeping a day—but spend an average of 8 hours 41 minutes on media devices." That is a ton of hours when you add up a month or even a week's worth.

I realize that the time I spend on devices can easily get out of hand, so I am cognizant of taking breaks and encouraging my family to do the same. Here are a few of my tactics:

- I often "detox" at least one day, a minimum of a few hours, on either Saturday or Sunday. I simply put my phone down (and leave it). I have actually begun leading Digital Rehab programs for people that want to learn to take baby steps to spend less time on their devices. Check out www.hotmessto-mindfulmom.com for details.
- We don't allow phones at family meals, and I have started leaving mine in the car when I eat out with my family.
- Our video gaming devices broke, and I am not fixing them. When kids come over for playdates, they have to find something else to do, preferably outside if the weather is nice.
- We have family game nights where we get out old-fashioned board games and spend some quality time together.
- I often put my phone into my purse when I am driving and use time at traffic lights to connect to my breath.
- I do not look at social media for at least thirty minutes before bed. Experts recommend turning technology off sixty minutes before bed. I like to read and watch shows on my iPad, so I am still working on that one!

Our kids do what we do much more than what we say, and technology is no exception. If we are on our phones and devices all

the time, we are showing our children that it is acceptable. When we take breaks, they notice, and may be more inclined to do the same. We have an amazing opportunity to model healthy habits around technology for our kids. Let's not waste it.

I challenge you to take one day and tally up how many minutes (or hours) you are on a device. The number may shock you! The average adult checks social media seventeen times a day. How do you fare against that statistic? Ask yourself if you feel good about your number and if there are ways you could reduce it. Have your kids do the same experiment, and talk about it as a family. What number feels good to each of you?

Come up with some ideas as a family of what you could do with the time saved by turning your devices off. Make a list of fun activities and hang it on the fridge as a reminder. They can be simple such as a bike ride or trip to the park, or more elaborate like a beach day that you have wanted to take forever. Cooking or baking is always a fun family activity—just remember, if you want to snap a pic of your kiddo covered in flour with a huge smile on their face, wait and post it later!

Baby steps really add up here. If it feels overwhelming to put your phone away for a whole hour on a weekend, try fifteen minutes to start and work up from there. It has to work for you, but once you step away for periods of time, I think you will really like it and want to do it more.

Another option is to offer some sort of reward system for time spent off technology or even make it an earned privilege. Here are a few ways to test that out in your own home:

- When kids spend thirty minutes reading, they can earn fifteen minutes of screen time.

- Kids can earn screen time by doing chores.
- Unlimited screen time one day a week by staying off the rest of the week.
- A certain time period of off-screen time earns a fun outing like an ice cream date or trip to the zoo.

Sometimes you don't know what will work for your family unless you try different things. This is one of those "date it before you marry it" situations. You can explain to your kids that you have an idea that you want to try in order to see how it works. If it doesn't end up working for your family, it is okay, and you can move on to Plan B. I would advise against getting too attached to any plan unless you know it feels good to you and you can manage it well. Adding something like a reward system is supposed to help you, not make your life a living hell trying to keep up with it.

As parents, being consistent is ingrained in us as the most necessary thing. There are many times, such as when we give a consequence, that I would say it is uber important. However, we only need to be consistent with the reward programs that work well for us. That is why I am seriously begging you to present this to your kids as an idea only at first. These are about trial and error. It is A-OK to tell our kids that a new idea was a bust. This is another opportunity to show our kids that it is okay to use our intuition and admit that we made a mistake.

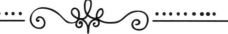

20

Tech Rules

Gotta Have 'Em!

"If you have never been hated by your child you have never been a parent."
—BETTE DAVIS

I was helping a coaching client to find the best time of day for her meditation practice. She knew she wanted morning, but she wanted it to be after she dropped her kids off at school. The problem was that she came home from drop-off starving, so she needed to stop and eat, which often led to other distractions. I asked her if she could eat with her kids before school, and she didn't feel that she could because there was too much to do, like feeding the dog, organizing lunches and snacks, and making breakfast for her preteen daughter.

I asked her if her daughter helped with a few simple tasks, like feeding the dog or organizing snacks, if it would free up time for her to make a quick smoothie. She said that yes, it would, but that her daughter was too busy on her phone in the morning before school to help, and she always came down late because she was on social media while she got ready.

I then asked her if she would be comfortable creating some boundaries and parameters around phone use, especially in the morning when it really seemed to get in the way. She was, and we decided on a few things together that she then communicated to her daughter and put into place. Here is what she put into action:

- Her daughter had to charge her phone in the kitchen. This way she couldn't stay up too late texting and being on social media, and she would have no distractions when getting ready for school.
- She and her daughter agreed on a time to be downstairs that didn't feel rushed. My client put an old-school alarm clock in her daughter's room so she could wake up on time without the alarm on her phone.
- Her daughter could have a few minutes to say hi to friends or do whatever was approved on her phone only after she had helped her mom feed the dog and get organized for the day.

Setting boundaries around technology can help to minimize the amount of fighting between parents and kids because expectations are clear and there simply isn't as much to argue about.

When one of my sons got his first phone, and the other one got an iPad, we all signed technology contracts. They stated:

"I understand that having a device is a privilege and a responsibility.

I respect that you love me and want to keep me safe online, and have my best interests at heart. With that we agree:

1. I understand that anything I write/text or put on social media is something that should be appropriate for my grandparents and teachers to see.

2. When my parents ask me to turn my device off, I will do so the first time they ask, or be prepared to hand the device to my parents.
3. I will only download apps and songs that are approved by my parents.
4. I understand that my parents have every right to look at my device, including texts.
5. I will not use my device during meals.
6. If I lose my device, I am responsible for replacing it."

I have family sharing on my phone and the kids' devices, so I have to approve all songs and apps that they download. There is another app that is really cool called OurPact, and it lets you schedule what times of day that your kids' devices will turn on, so you have complete control over their use. You can set it to only turn on on the weekends, or only for thirty minutes after school as a short break before homework, for example.

I decided to go with the idea that they must turn them off when I ask because I liked the flexibility that it offered. That's why I didn't include a time limit in our contract. If I tell them that they have thirty minutes a day or sixty minutes a day, they will hound me until they get to use each and every one of them. Some days don't allow for device time because we are hopping from school to sports and then finishing homework and bedtime. That's just how it goes. Some days we have a lot more down time and it doesn't bother me that they are on their device or watching TV for a bit longer because it all balances out. As a working mom, there are days the kids don't have school and I have to see clients, so they may be on it a bit more than I would like. I just make sure that doesn't happen too often, but selfishly at times, their devices make my life easier!

I know that a lot of people have a rule stating no technology during the week. That is definitely one way to go. I don't mind the kids winding down before bed with a twenty-minute show after a long day if there is time. As I said, there isn't time every single night. I tend to be a little more go-with-the-flow in this area, but there are some general rules that I think are good, like the ones I included in our contract.

Contracts and comfort levels are personal, and will vary from family to family. I also told my kids that contracts can be evaluated and updated based on what is working and what isn't. These were simply our starting point.

Devices are not in the vicinity of homework or meals. My husband and I follow the same rule about mealtimes too, since it helps us all to be more present, to connect, and it gives us a chance to model the behavior we want our kids to have.

I have also talked to my preteen at length about "likes." He downloaded the social media app Instagram and immediately became enamored with getting likes on posts, and I could see the slippery slope we were on. We had a long talk about likes, and I explained to him that we should never value our self-worth or self-esteem on how many likes we get. We have to feel good about the choices we make and what we partake in no matter what kind of attention we get about it from others. Now he'll say to me, "Mom, I got twenty likes on my post, but I know it doesn't change how I feel about myself." I think the message is starting to sink in!

Contracts are also wonderful tools to use for homework, chores, or time spent out with friends once your kids hit the preteen and teen years.

One of my mentors, parenting expert Susan Epstein, LCSW, of www.parentingpowers.com, has a contract she gives to her parent

clients to use when their preteens and teens go out with friends un-supervised that I think is brilliant. That may seem like a long way off for some of you reading, but it will be here before you know it! Since we are focusing on kids up to twelve, not everything will apply, but it is always good to see what we need to be aware of down the line. For now, take the pieces that make sense. It states:

"I know that going out with my friends without parental super-vision is a privilege. I respect that you love me and want to keep me safe. You respect that I am no longer a small child and want the privi-lege of going out to places with my friends without your supervision. With that in mind, we agree:

1. I will always tell you where I am going to be, who I am going to be with, and what I am going to be doing.
2. If I am going to be at a friend's house, I will share the address and phone number with you, and the cell phone number of a parent.
3. My curfew is _____. This can be negotiated for both of us. My curfew means I am inside my home.
4. I understand I must speak to you as soon as I come home.
5. I will call or text and ask your permission if my plans have changed, and will not go anywhere without checking with you first.
6. I understand that you have the right and responsibility to check up on me not only when you feel the need, but from time to time to keep me safe. I will respond, because when I don't respond you imagine the worst, and you want to be sure I am safe.
7. I will respect the limits and guidelines set forth by my friend's parents.

8. I agree that if I am unable to keep up with my responsibilities, such as my schoolwork and chores, I can lose the privilege of going out with friends.

9. I understand that I can call you at any time if I feel threatened or unsafe when I am out with my friends. I will not have consequences for pulling myself out of a bad situation. Our code word if I need you to get me but I don't feel comfortable saying why in front of my friends is _____.

10. The consequences for not following through with these guidelines on going out with friends unsupervised are:

- _____
- _____
- _____

I feel really old when I hear about a new social media app these days. My first thought is "Another thing to learn!" I feel really happy and fulfilled with the few social media, channels I am on, and I truly don't have the desire to add more to my repertoire because I am always struggling to spend less time online, not more! However, when our kids are on social media, we have no choice but to get on whatever the hip new platform is so that we can follow them. That may be all we do on it, but we need to have an account to follow them.

Our kids need to understand that we give them the privilege of social media in conjunction with the responsibility of being safe and making good choices. It is also our responsibility as parents to be monitoring their online behavior. Our kids should know that we will be intermittently popping onto their channels to be sure everything looks kosher. Our goal isn't to embarrass them by commenting and necessarily joining the conversation they are having with their friends, in fact I don't recommend that, but our job is to keep them

safe. Keeping them safe means that we can ask questions about their online friends.

We are gearing this conversation to our kids that are twelve and younger right now, so there is a very high likelihood that you will know every single friend they have, and most likely they are on one, maybe two social media channels, at most. We are setting the groundwork and ground rules for open lines of communication in the future, pertaining to social media and appropriate online behavior.

At eleven, my son is only allowed to accept friend requests from people that we both know, but as he gets older and meets more people through activities and athletics, I know that will change. The fact that I can ask who they are won't!

I am the product of divorced parents who had different rules. Now that I am a parent, I don't think they had enough rules, which is why I don't want my kids doing anything that I did growing up. Those stories will most likely not make it into any of my books!

I believe that it is very important for parents—regardless of whether they are unmarried, married, separated, or divorced—to be on the same page when it comes to rules in general, including rules surrounding technology and social media. Parents must portray a united front, and should come up with tech rules together and uphold the same consequences when rules are broken.

I am not divorced, but I can imagine that agreeing on rules may be strained and uncomfortable. My parents hardly spoke to each other after their divorce and they definitely didn't confer on rules for my sisters and I. With my perspective as a parent, I can now see how beneficial that would have been for me as a preteen and teenager. If it is at all possible, I encourage you to put it on your radar and attempt. As far as parents that are still married and live together, no excuses!

21

Transition Tactics

Ten Minutes Can Turn Your Morning Around!

"If you have told your child a thousand times and he still does not understand, then it is not the child who is the slow learner."

—WALTER BARBIE

I don't know about you, but we start each school year with a fresh attitude and dedication and enthusiasm for the rules around our morning routines.

The mornings during summer vacation that my kids are not at overnight camp are the complete antithesis of our weekday schedule and are *way* more relaxed and chill. My kids wake up with their own body clock, which is still earlier than I would like, and watch TV. Breakfast may be around 9:00 a.m., followed by a game of cards, and then finally getting dressed around 10:00 a.m. A very far cry from a school day!

So when it is time to head back to school, we always have a quick family meeting to discuss expectations, responsibilities, and schedules.

I typically get up between 5:45 and 6:00 a.m. for my own self-care routine, which I described in detail earlier. The kids set an alarm and are responsible for being dressed and downstairs at 7:00 a.m. ready to start the day. I eat breakfast with the kids and attend to any last-minute additions to their lunches, which have typically been prepared the night before. By 7:30 a.m. when we need to walk out the door, the kids are responsible for brushing their teeth and packing snacks and lunches in their backpacks, as well as any special things that needs to go to school that day such as a project that's due.

This routine runs like clockwork until about March or April of the school year. That's when things often begin to slip and the routine starts closer to 7:10 a.m. Then it feels like there is a bit of a mad rush to get it all done by 7:30 a.m. This is when it becomes glaringly obvious how much of a difference ten minutes can make.

When I am out of town my husband has a different routine with the kids altogether. They get downstairs at 6:50 a.m., and there is never a mad dash. They head out at 7:20 a.m. and the kids are nearly the first at school, which they like. So guess what I decided to try when I got home and heard about this amazing new system? Yup, new times, and I loved it. I didn't eat standing at the counter, I actually sat down at the table with my kids and started the day feeling calmer and more connected. Ten minutes began to equate to calm and peace in our mornings.

This ten-minute rule began to spill over into other areas of our lives as well. I find that one of my kids isn't great with transitions if he is rushed. If I say last minute, "Sweetie, let's go right now," he may whine and complain that he isn't ready. But if I make sure he knows that we have to leave in ten minutes, he has time to mentally prepare for the transition, and our departure goes much smoother.

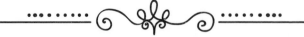

Many tasks can be done in ten minutes, and lots of things end up taking about ten minutes longer than you think they will. For this reason, I am planning for more transitions in my calendar instead of feeling like I am constantly rushed.

Where can you give yourself an extra ten minutes in your day? Here are some times when it can be especially helpful:

- Getting ready in the morning.
- Heading out to an activity when traffic may be bad.
- Starting the kids' bedtime routine ten minutes earlier so lights actually go out at the time you want.
- Prepping for dinner.
- Not starting a new task ten minutes before you need to walk out the door so you can collect everything you need for errands or a work day.

Since the flow of the household starts with me and my attitude and preparation, I have found that the more time and space I give myself to eliminate the feeling of rushing, which leads to anxiety and stress, the better mood I am in. The better mood I am in, the better I can deal with unexpected emergencies, sibling bickering, and tasks on my to-do list. When I try to pack too many things into my day, that is when I feel out of control and triggered. I have learned this the hard way! I encourage you to give yourself and your kids a little more breathing room. Ten minutes really can make all the difference.

If mornings feel hard for you, try to remember your "why" and how much smoother they go when you give yourself a cushion. Resist hitting the snooze button and take just a split second to weigh how your morning will go if you hit snooze and then feel rushed

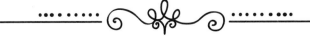

instead of getting up and moving into your day feeling calm and in control.

I tell people all the time that it is just hard to get up in the morning in general. It isn't harder to get up ten minutes earlier. Who wants to leave their warm, cozy bed to face the cold floor? I don't! But it isn't any easier ten minutes later. What I have realized as well is that when I do snooze I don't go back to sleep. I lie there thinking of how I am going to feel rushed, berating myself for wasting precious time that could be useful, and wishing that I had just gotten up. Sounds like heaven, doesn't it? Totally not worth it.

Bottom line—ten minutes is no biggie in the grand scheme of your morning. Just get up!

22

Prioritize Your Partner

The early date before the date

"I want the kind of marriage that makes my kids want to get married."
—EMILY WIERENGA

My husband and I have always prioritized our relationship and spending quality time together, even after we had kids. So much of our family life revolves around our boys, but we both feel strongly about keeping our connection as partners and spouses.

As the byproduct of divorced parents, I know firsthand how important the strength of a marriage is to the success of the family overall. I wasn't surprised when my parents said they were getting divorced. Even as a young girl of eleven, I was perceptive enough to see that even though they didn't fight, they never truly seemed connected.

It is unrealistic to think that parents will never disagree or occasionally fight. If your kids are going to see you argue, aim to be conscious of your language and tone. Kids pick up on your energy.

If they do see you argue, let them see you make up. They probably won't be privy to the entire conversation, but let them hear you say the words "I'm sorry" and give a hug. It's important for children to understand that we will have moments of frustration with people that we love, but we work through it and come back together. This is important modeling.

I had a lot of insecurities as a child. Heck, a few (or more accurately, many) of them followed me into adulthood, and although I have processed many of them, I am still working through a few. I can't blame everything on my parents, nor would I ever give anyone that much responsibility to shoulder for me, but I do think that the more kids see teamwork amongst their parents, the better. This goes for all parents, married or divorced.

When kids witness open lines of communication and respect between their parents they feel more secure, and it feels safe to be a kid. I never felt secure as a child. I remember being eight years old and asking if we had health insurance.

I had a funny conversation with my twin sister recently. I was staying with her, and one of the kids was asking for something or other that they needed for school, and my sister said, "Sure, I'll get it." I looked at her and wondered out loud what it would be like to feel so secure growing up and knowing that all your needs were going to be met, no problem. I feel blessed and grateful that my kids don't have the same kinds of worries that I did as a child. I was forced to grow up way too fast.

I am a very affectionate person. I remember my uncle once told me that he had never seen someone kiss their kids as much as me. I took it as a compliment!

Fortunately, my husband is the perfect match for me on the snuggle scale. He likes to hold hands, hug, and cuddle. Between him,

my kids, and my dogs, I am often found snuggling someone. I like that my kids see that we are connected in this way.

Not everyone likes to be as affectionate, and it certainly isn't a prerequisite to a happy marriage by any means, but I think finding a close match on the snuggle scale can be a nice bonus. If one partner loves to snuggle, and one hates it, there could be disappointment, frustration, or resentment stewing. Open lines of communication and telling our partner what we need at certain times can really combat these issues, though. Our partners aren't mind readers! We may need to tell them straight up, "I had a hard day, and I really need a hug."

Saturday night "date night" has always been a part of our routine. We resumed our Saturday nights out when my first son was three weeks old and again when my second was two weeks. I had a reliable babysitter that I totally trusted, and although some people may think that it's nuts to leave a baby with a sitter that early, I was ready, especially because I didn't breastfeed so I didn't have to be home with my boobs in order to feed my babies.

I had actually planned on breastfeeding, but unfortunately I had complications with it, and it didn't go as I had hoped. I released all guilt surrounding breastfeeding, deciding that my babies would be as happy as I was. However, for any of you new moms who can't get away so easily, I encourage you to find a way to carve out some time for yourselves, even if that just means dressing up for a date night in the kitchen while the baby is sleeping or getting a sitter for an hour while you and your hubby go for an ice cream.

Because my husband and I were able to get out for a little bit longer, many of our Saturday nights out included plans with other couples and parent friends who were also looking for a grown-up night away from baby food and diapers. We all got dressed up, put

on makeup, and had to keep our cell phones on the table in case our sitter needed us. But how many times have you gone to dinner with a group of friends and all the women sit on one end of the table and the men on the other? That kept happening, so by the time we got home after dinner my husband and I hadn't said two words to each other. We were exhausted by that point, and had to get up at 5:00 a.m. with my early-rising son, so there was no talking before bed. To combat the lack of interaction on nights out with friends, we started doing "pre-dates."

Our sitters now come at least an hour earlier than we need them to so that Mark and I can do something alone before we meet friends. Sometimes we go to Starbucks, sometimes we have a drink at the bar where we are meeting people, sometimes we work out together and shower at the gym. A favorite is also going to get foot massages together. It truly doesn't matter what we do, as long as we are alone. It is the perfect way for us to balance alone and social time.

Now that the kids are older, our weekly nights out have dwindled to about twice a month. Our kids may be invited to a party with us, they may have a baseball tournament with night games, or sometimes we just like to include them now that they are older and so much more fun on a Saturday night out. We still need date nights and social time, but our kids get so excited for weekend nights out with us, and we love it, too. Pretty soon they will be ditching us for their friends, so we want to be with them as much as we can!

Next time you plan a night out with friends, organize a "pre-date" and see how it feels. Do you and your partner feel more connected? If so, make it a part of your date night routine.

23

Check Yourself Before You Wreck Yourself

Don't react . . . respond!

"If you wouldn't say it to a friend, don't say it to yourself."
—JANE TRAVIS

This. Is. A. Game-Changer.

I would say this has been the biggest change in me—as a mom and a person—along my entire journey. I don't know if anyone would have described me as a yeller, but I definitely lost my patience quite easily, which has been a pattern I have worked on since childhood. Growing up, I was a foot-stomper. If I didn't get my way or was pissed off at someone in my family, I would cross my arms and stomp my feet. I am still haunted by the memories of my entire family standing up around the dining room table and doing it at the same time as me just to show me how silly I looked. Very silly indeed. I can admit that as an adult I have stamped my foot a time

or two, without even realizing, and my husband will ask me, "Did you just stomp your foot?" And I can't help but laugh. Old habits die hard.

Fortunately, I have found another way to live these days, which is much more socially acceptable and enjoyable, too. These days I try to check myself before I wreck myself.

The name of the game is awareness. Since I practice this constantly I can get a bit ahead of my emotions, and I can feel them coming on; in the olden days I would go from zero to sixty, and all of a sudden I'd lost complete control of myself. Now, I can usually feel my emotions escalating and use a tool from my toolbox to help calm me down before I lose it. There are times where I don't quite catch myself, but by coming back to my breath or using another part of my trigger plan, I can recover much, much faster.

My trigger plan consists of:

- Doing a quick, one-minute meditation.
- Pausing and making myself a cup of tea.
- Getting into nature, even for just a minute or two on my back porch.
- Lying on the floor and snuggling with my dogs.

For others it may be connecting with a friend, exercising, or taking a bath. There is no right or wrong, simply what works for you. The key is actually *using* your trigger plan. The more you use it, the more habitual it gets, and the more it can help you in times of actual stress.

My goal is to *pause, reflect,* and *choose.*

This is one area where the more modeling we do for our kids, the better. Because my kids see me pause to breathe when I feel trig-

gered or stressed, it is easier for me to talk to them about doing it themselves. This is a prime example of teaching our kids through our own actions rather than talking to them like Charlie Brown's teacher, when all they hear is "whah, whah, whah, whah, whah."

I was tested by my ten-year-old, and it ended up being the perfect time to have a conversation about this very topic. One afternoon he was being disrespectful, which he knows is not tolerated in our home. I excused him to his room and told him that he was welcome to come back down anytime he was ready to alter his tone. He knows that is code for take a few minutes to breathe and chill out.

My kids have seen me pause in the middle of many situations to take a few nice, long deep breaths, and because I have created an environment in our home where that is a normal response, they will often pause to breathe too when they feel overwhelmed or upset. *The keyword is "often."* My son did not do that in this case and needed some downtime to regroup.

Later that evening as I was tucking my son into bed, he apologized for his disrespectful tone. Because he brought it up, I jumped on the chance to talk about it, especially since bedtime is when my son really opens up and shares with me. I asked him if he could tell that he was feeling agitated and getting triggered, and he said yes. I then told him one of my favorite lines: "Babe, you gotta check yourself before you wreck yourself."

I explained that awareness is the key in any situation. When you feel your emotions escalating, you need to check in. I explain this as the "yums" and the "yucks." When we are feeling sad or anxious, we may have feelings in our body like a pit in our stomach, a headache, or it feels harder to breathe and our body feels tight. These are really yucky feelings and we feel them when we are triggered. Something happens in our environment, and a feeling arises in our body. I ex-

plained to my son that when he's feeling the yucks, he needs to check in with his body to figure out what will make him feel better. What are you needing in that moment? How can you get back to center? Do you need to breathe? Do you need to excuse yourself? Do you need to talk? Do you need a hug?

Just like us, it can be difficult for our children to handle stress in the moment. When they are all riled up, it can be hard for them to even think about how they can help themselves. Talking to your kids when they are calm to help them make a list of three or four things that always make them feel better is a great plan. Once you come up with a list together, you can post it in a prominent place like the fridge or in their room for them to refer to when they feel themselves beginning to lose control of their emotions. The list can have things on it like:

- Spending time with my pet.
- Reading a book.
- Coloring.
- Doing a crossword puzzle.
- Talking to Mom or Dad.
- Collecting leaves from outside.
- Organizing trading cards.
- A card with "1, 2, 3" written on it so they can remember to match their inhale and exhale to a count of three.
- Special pictures that make them feel calm and happy.
- A journal to write out their feelings.

You can even help your kids make a special bag that they can easily grab when they feel triggered and stressed with all the materials they need to carry out their trigger plan, like coloring books and markers, a book, or a journal.

One thing I love about the concept of a trigger plan for kids is that it creates a language that makes sense to both parents and kids. In a particularly yuck moment, kids will probably not be up for a big conversation about how to get out of their funk. Instead, when they (or you) start to notice the physical trigger signs, they have a way to self-soothe and calm down until they are ready to talk about what's wrong.

Reading the signals of our bodies is like learning a new language. We have to practice and really pay attention. Once we learn how our body communicates with us, it gets a lot easier to use these signals to make decisions. Think about how empowering this is for kids! They have a built-in GPS system that can help them make good choices. I wish I understood this concept when I was growing up. I would have made better choices for sure!

I've heard so many parents with kids in high school and college tell me, "Bigger kids equal bigger problems." It's really true when you think about what could potentially be coming down the line like cigarettes, alcohol, drugs, and sex. I start sweating just typing the words! We don't do ourselves or our kids any favors by burying our heads in the sand. That is why open lines of communication when kids are learning to make choices at a young age are so important. We have the opportunity to guide them and teach them how to make choices that feel good to them while they are young. If they learn to say no when a situation doesn't feel right at a young age, saying no to these bigger things when dealing with peer pressure may not feel quite as hard. We can help them bring awareness to themselves so they can check before they wreck.

Sometimes, though, no matter how much you work with your kids on building a toolkit to stay calm, they're going to lose it. When your kids are throwing a temper tantrum, that's when it's more important than ever to remember your own trigger plan.

Every time I give my kids a consequence during an outburst or occasional disrespectful backtalk, I regret it. When I haven't taken the time to calmly think about what makes the most sense, I inevitably say something, realize that it wasn't really the consequence I wanted to give, and then am forced to stick to it, basically punishing myself.

There are certain times when natural consequences are obvious, like when my son used to completely lose his cool if he wasn't winning during a family basketball game on the driveway. We talked to him many times regarding the right times to be competitive and the right times to just have a little fun. It got to the point that if he cried and threw a fit, he was excused from the game. Automatically. There was no better natural consequence than that.

But then there are other situations where I want to confer with my husband or take some time to think, so I'll tell my kids just that. I want to talk to their dad, or I need time to think about the best way to proceed. I am then modeling for them that it is okay to calm down from a situation and take time to think about how you want to proceed. It is also important that they see their parents as a united front, and not just one as the "bad guy" always doling out the punishments.

When my kids do fall apart, I try my best to remember that they feel safe enough and loved enough with me to do it. They have to hold it together at school, and with friends, and on the sports field. Sometimes they just need to cry and move that emotion around. Haven't you ever felt better after a good cry? I have! But there are ways to do it that are okay and ways that aren't, and those boundaries do need to be taught. Verbalizing frustration is perfectly okay. Throwing things around the house is not.

24

The Best Way to
Get Your Kids' Attention
You can get them to listen!

"Yelling silences your message. Speak quietly so your children can hear your words instead of just your voice."

—L.R. KNOST

I will never forget the day that my son screamed "Jesus Christ" out of frustration in a public place. I was mortified, mostly because he sounded like me.

He was repeating a very inappropriate, possibly offensive phrase that I had been saying when I was frustrated, and hearing it out of his mouth I learned firsthand just how bad I sounded. There was no question that he had learned it from me. So yes, it was embarrassing, but mostly because I couldn't look around and say, "Whose kid is that anyway?" I had no choice but to take responsibility for my own actions and vocabulary.

Our children are our mirrors, for the good and the bad. Their manners reflect the ones taught at home, and their sometimes off-color language gives you a glimpse into what is being said at home, too. It works both ways!

Most parents I know feel like their kids don't listen to them, or at least not the first, second, or third time they ask them to do something. I wonder, is this another way that they are mirroring us?

My New Year's resolution every single year is to stop interrupting others when they are speaking. Interrupting others is a horrible habit that I have, and I know it. I feel embarrassed when I do it, and I have become super aware and can now catch myself in the act. It comes from a place of excitement and passion, but it still comes off as rude.

In my meditation teacher training, we learned how to "listen with love," and my ears really perked up during this lesson. This was information I desperately needed, as I deeply wanted to improve in this area. When you listen with love you are fully present to what the other person is saying, without half-listening and simultaneously formulating your response in your head. When you truly listen, you are able to connect to the speaker's emotions and really understand where they are coming from. This can also be called active listening. I wonder how often we listen to our kids this way. When your kids talk, are you:

- Making eye contact with them?
- Maintaining presence?
- Letting them finish their sentences without being interrupted?
- Making sure they feel heard?

Modeling good listening skills for our kids shows them the way we want them to listen to us. Here are a few things that have really

worked for my own family and also for my clients in terms of getting kids to listen. I call them my ninja mom tricks:

Make eye contact when you ask your kids to do something

Yelling at your kids from the kitchen that it is time to get shoes on while their eyes are glued to the television is simply not going to end well. Taking the extra step to get in front of your kids and look them in the eye when you are speaking to them will really pay off and cut down on frustration on both ends.

Have them repeat back the request

This has really been a game changer with my own kids, and it takes away the excuse they try to use with me all the time: "I didn't hear you."

When I ask my kids to do something I have them immediately repeat it back to me. If I say, "We are leaving in two minutes, please get on your shoes," they must repeat back to me, "We are leaving in two minutes and we have to get our shoes on." If I can tell they are not 100 percent with me, I will ask them, "What is happening in two minutes?" They say, "We are leaving." I ask, "What do you need to do?" They answer, "Put on our shoes."

It sounds really juvenile and excessive, but it works like magic. I am crystal clear, and they know exactly what my expectations are.

Whisper

Yelling doesn't get my kids to do what I want, and it makes me feel like a crappy mom. Instead, I try to whisper. For some reason when I

speak really quietly, they hang on every word. Speaking really quietly also helps to keep me calm. I hate yelling. I feel horrible and it never ends up accomplishing what I want, and I end up just wishing for a do-over. As the parents, we need to remain calm no matter what. Our kids need to see us as cool, calm, and collected, no matter how they try to rile us. This is where your trigger plan and lots of deep breathing can really come in handy.

Take a time out

When I feel myself begin to lose control and become really triggered around my kids, I often decide it is best for me to take a break from the situation so that I can breathe and collect myself. I may also need to gather my thoughts and determine the best way to respond to my kids instead of reacting in a way I will regret, or throwing out some consequence that doesn't feel right ten minutes later that we are both stuck with. When I say "Mom needs a time out" and walk in the other room, my kids know when I walk back in I mean business, and this usually gets their full attention.

When my kids aren't listening, it is ordinarily because I am not making eye contact with them and being sure they heard me by having them repeat back the request. This sometimes happens if I get lazy, and then I have nobody to be mad at besides myself, but it is a great reminder to recommit to my mindful habits.

Occasionally technology can get in the way of my kids listening. As I mentioned before, it is part of our technology contract that they must turn off their devices the first time I ask them to, or they must hand them over. I know as we get into the teenage years this may become more of a battle, but I do feel like I am laying the groundwork now as best I can.

There are also times that I have to level with my kids no-holds-barred. If I am not feeling well, or am beyond exhausted after a super long day, I let them know what is going on. I am not afraid for them to see me in this vulnerable state. I will tell them that I am completely exhausted, and I need serious, extra-special help and cooperation.

It is important that our kids see and understand that we don't have it together every minute of every day. That doesn't mean we are screaming and yelling like crazy (because I won't ever advocate that!), but maybe our energy is low, or maybe we got sad news, or maybe we had a crappy day at work and we just need an easy night.

Vulnerability is okay. If we put on a brave face all the time, we aren't teaching our kids to be honest about their own feelings and emotions. If they only see our life as perfectly pulled together, will they think they are normal on days when they feel a bit sad or low-energy themselves? Because it will happen eventually. Even though we don't want to think of our sweet little pea pods as anything but happy, there will be a day when they won't feel happy. And all feelings are okay. Just because we are sad one day doesn't mean we are sad people. Just because we are in a bad mood one day doesn't mean we are moody all the time. We don't have to attach to our emotions in that way. Emotions are something to be experienced in the moment, not something that will dictate all our days going forward.

If we are brave enough to be honest with our kids about how we are feeling on occasion, we have a beautiful opportunity to help them develop empathy. Have you ever been sad and one of your kids drew you a picture to make you feel better and in turn you thought they were as sweet as cotton candy? If you hadn't expressed your sadness, they wouldn't have had the opportunity to do something so heartfelt and loving.

I had to get over wanting to shelter my kids from everything that wasn't sunshine and roses because I wasn't helping them grow as people. They have seen me cry happy tears every time they are on a stage at school or when they show kindness to a friend, but they have also occasionally seen me cry out of sadness.

Every day isn't awesome. I want my kids to have realistic expectations about that, or life will feel really, really hard as they grow. They will learn resilience from this. They will practice using their trigger plans because of it. They will see that they can't control everything that happens to them in life, but they can control how they react to it.

If you ask most parents what they want for their kids in life, an overwhelming number of them will say, "I want my child to be happy." But what does that mean? Does that mean I want life to be perfect so they don't ever have to deal with adversity or being hurt? I want my kids to be able to raise themselves up from challenges with their positive attitude and with determination to be the best they can be. I want my kids to see that life can be challenging but they are strong, and they will make it through. I want my kids to understand that not everyone will be nice, and they will witness horrible things being said, but that they should always choose to be kind even if that means walking away from people who don't hold the same standard. I want them to have the tools they need to succeed in life—if I had to pick five I would choose positivity, confidence, a kind heart, strength of character, and an unwavering connection to their intuition. What would you pick for your five?

25

Get Your Kids on Your Team

Works every time

"There will be so many times you feel like you've failed. But in the eyes, heart, and mind of your child, you are Super Mom."

—STEPHANIE PRECOURT

Many things in life require two people: marriage, ballroom dancing, singing a duet, competing in "The Amazing Race," and being a twin. The parent/child combination is a dynamic duo that sometimes takes my breath away. I almost didn't get it until I had my own kids. I remember looking at my mom when I was holding my newborn, and I asked her, "You love me *this* much?" I mean, I always knew my parents loved me, but I couldn't grasp just how much until I was a mother myself.

I have always been a big collaborator. I love connecting, sharing creative ideas, and working toward a common goal. I didn't get to be captain of my cheerleading team in high school because I was the best on the team, but because I was inclusive and I got shit done.

Being part of a team feels good to me, so I decided to carry that mentality into my family life as well. Just call us Team Katz! My boys are sports fanatics so they understand what it feels like to be a valued member of a team and how to carry your weight. The language around being a team was something they could relate to as soon as they swung their first bat.

If your kids have never been part of a team, this is a great opportunity to explain how teams work and why it is important for everyone to contribute to the team's success. Learning to work with others is a life skill that needs to be developed for a successful career as a human being, and a family team can be the perfect way to start!

Using the team mentality and framework puts a positive spin on things that have to get done in real life. Instead of something being one person's responsibility, it feels more fun and cohesive for it to be a family team's responsibility.

My kids have heard many a mommy motivational speech begin with, "Hey guys, I need you on my team. You ready?" I do this because it works. This book focuses on kids between ages five and twelve; I am not suggesting that this will work with teenagers, but younger kids still want to please you and have fun with you. That being said, the closer the bonds with our kids when they are young, the better chance we can keep that closeness as they grow into teenagers. We want to foster that connection, communication, and trust, so we can keep it going. Accomplishing tasks as a team allows for collaboration and creates more opportunities to work side by side with your kids, which may encourage them to open up. Just like some kids feel more comfortable opening up when riding in the car, others feel more comfortable when they have something to do with their hands and aren't eye to eye with you. Sometimes they just want to vent in an environment that doesn't feel like a "talk," or they might feel slightly

embarrassed to admit something, and working side by side can add another layer of comfort and is a way to encourage them to open up.

There are several ways and times when the team mentality is really helpful. Great times to foster teamwork in your house is:

Bedtime

Every mom knows what it feels like to dread bedtime at the end of the day. Your eyes are burning, you have done a mountain of dishes, and you just want to curl up with your remote and binge watch your favorite show. Yes, the snuggles and kisses right at tuck-in time are the reward for all your hard work the past twelve-plus hours, but the journey from the kitchen to the kids' rooms by way of the bathroom sometimes feels downright daunting.

On nights when I just feel D-O-N-E and I want bedtime to run smooth as silk, I bust out my Team Katz speech. I get the kids all pumped up and tell them that bedtime is going to be a team effort. I usually give two or three directions, then tell them there is a time limit, and I set the microwave timer. So the spiel would go something like this, "Guys, let's make bedtime extra fun tonight by being a team and seeing how fast we can do it when we all work together. Let's see if we can do it in seven minutes!" (This would be a night that they occasionally skip a shower. If they need to shower, I would up the time to maybe twenty minutes.) If your kids are younger, you would have to go upstairs with them and maybe set a timer on your watch to see how fast they can get ready for bed.

There could also be a reward. For example, if they do it in a certain amount of time, they get an extra book before bed, a five-minute back tickle, or two extra songs—whatever you think would motivate them. Older kids may like an extra ten minutes to read or

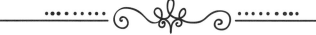

a game of cards on their bed. The rewards allow you to spend a few extra minutes enjoying your kids rather than using all the time to ask them ten times to get ready for bed.

Making dinner/setting the table

Teamwork setting the table or helping to prep for dinner may just leave enough time to play a game before you eat or shoot some hoops outside. Kids usually love to help prepare meals, and maybe they get a fun little appetizer while they help.

I love when my kids help me in the kitchen because they usually munch on the veggies they cut, but it is also a time when great conversations can take place about the day, school, and friends. This is yet another chance for your kids to open up to you while everyone works side by side, and it doesn't feel like you are grilling them for info.

Get the kids on your team by telling them that dinner will get done faster so there is time to do _____ before you eat.

During travel

A few things that really scare me are airports, gas stations, and train stations. I get nervous any time I am somewhere that a stranger could potentially kidnap my kid and take them far away from me quickly. I know this could certainly happen anywhere, but places of travel have just always had me on extra-high alert.

Ever since my kids were little, I have used the team analogy when traveling. Everyone has a job to do. Mine is to watch the boys, and the boys' job is to stay close to me. They get a little reminder on the way and as we walk in the door of one of these places.

Heading out the door

It can be overwhelming enough to get out the door alone. Did you eat? Do you have your phone? Car keys? Is the sleep out of your eyes? Adding kids into the mix can send a mom over the edge if the kids don't help out because there are lots more questions. Did the kids eat? Are lunches packed? Are they wearing sneakers on PE days? Is homework in the backpack? Is the soccer stuff packed for after school? It is a *lot!*

Acting as a team can truly be a game changer if you make a plan and let your kids know how important their help is. We've all heard that there is no "I" in team, and this includes family teams. It takes everyone to pull together. Maybe you dole out jobs each morning, or maybe there is a list on the fridge of what everyone is responsible for. Try it different ways and see what works for your family.

Doing chores

Chores get done much quicker when the family works together. Mom shouldn't be the only one picking up! There are so many ways to divvy up responsibilities like:

- Making beds
- Vacuuming
- Unloading the dishwasher
- Laundry
- Feeding and walking pets

There are as many ways to divide up chores as there are actual tasks! Some families like to keep a chart and take turns each week. Others let the kids negotiate with each other and trade. It doesn't

matter at all, as long as the chores get done and everyone works as a team.

So, there is one obvious question that arises here: What if your kids aren't into it? What if no matter how fun you make it sound, and no matter how positive you are, when you try to get them on your team they look at you like you have two heads? With young kids, it is unlikely, but not out of the question. It could be an off day, or your kids could be tired and would much rather be playing a video game.

I would explain that the chores, going to bed, or heading out the door is not optional. Whatever it is needs to happen, and will happen, but there is a way that it can be enjoyable to do it together or a way that it can stink, and it is up to them. The good news is that you are together and can work to get past the task quickly and onto the fun if everyone chips in. Otherwise it will take longer and drag out. The natural consequence is that the longer the task takes, the less time there is for fun.

There are times I have had to level with my kids and explain to them that I am really, really tired, and I honestly just need their help. These are the times that I am so pooped that I don't know how I will make it to my own bedtime, and since I don't feel that way often, my kids usually step up to the plate when I explain how I feel. The key is not to yell, but to calmly explain how you are feeling, and try to relate it to how they feel sometimes by saying something like, "You know how you felt after your soccer game when you ran and ran and then crashed in the car? I am tired like that, but I can't get rest until dinner is made and the dishes are done and you are in bed. I really need you to hop on my team and be my helper to get everything accomplished. It would mean a lot and would really help me. Maybe we can even get done in time to relax and watch a show on the couch together or have some extra snuggles before bed." Who can resist that?

26

Systems That Work

Set yourself up for success

"If you want your children to improve, let them overhear the nice things you say about them to others."

—HAIM GINOTT

I have never found that fly-by-the-seat-of-my-pants motherhood worked for me. From everything you have read so far, that is probably pretty obvious! Even though I have chilled out in many ways, I still like to plan, and I flat-out adore lists.

One night I was tucking my older son in, and I saw a note that he had written reminding himself of what to do when he woke up in the morning. I said to myself, "That's my kid!"

My older son is 100% percent a reflection of me, and my younger one is every ounce my husband. It is really amazing how it happened like that. Sometimes I want to just tell my older son "Sorry" for a few of the idiosyncrasies he got from me. My husband can't relate to all of them, but I can. I know *just* where he is coming from.

For example, he takes after me when he writes everything down and when I remind him of something he asks me to make him a note. He likes to know "the plan," and needs a combination of social and alone time. He is really hard on himself, like I used to be before I adopted an attitude of self-compassion, which I hope that I can help him foster.

Kids crave consistency and routine because it makes them feel safe and secure. I can even relate to that as an adult! There are tons of ways that you can set up systems in your home with lists so that you and the kids know just what to do and when. Lists also empower kids and give them independence. They don't have to ask you about every move they make because they understand what is expected of them and can become responsible for it.

The hardest part of parenting so far for me has been giving my kids more independence and autonomy. If I am being brutally honest, it feels nice to be needed, and sometimes it is easier to just do things myself. It is certainly faster and neater most times! But I am not doing my kids any favors by stripping them of the chance to make choices and have responsibility. It got to the point that I could see myself crippling them at times, and I realized that this was really an area for me to grow. I began giving them more responsibility around the house with things like:

- Loading and unloading the dishwasher.
- Packing and unpacking for sleepovers.
- Helping to cut vegetables for dinner.
- Feeding the dogs.
- Packing their own snacks for school.
- Being in charge of their morning allergy medicine.

They can often do so much more than we give them credit for or expect them to do. I remember the morning that my son, at eight

years old, came downstairs early and made breakfast for himself and his brother, lined up their shoes and backpacks, poured the allergy medicine, and put toothpaste on their toothbrushes and had them waiting for after breakfast. At that point it was pretty apparent what he was capable of and that I was holding him back. My next thought was that I needed to teach him how to make my chai tea misto and have it waiting for me next time!

Then there are the times that you let them grow up while simultaneously feeling like you need a paper bag to breathe into so you don't hyperventilate. That was me the first time I let my son ride his bike around the block with a neighbor. I wasn't so sure about it, but he looked at me and said, "Mom, I'm ready!" so what was I to do? He wasn't going to be alone, and he really wanted to try.

As I watched him turn off our street I felt my chest constrict and my breath became short. It sounds ridiculous now, but at the time it felt like a piece of my heart just left the street. I immediately called my husband at work and told him that maybe I made the wrong choice. Maybe it was too soon. I wondered if I should run and follow them. My husband talked me off the ledge, and a few minutes later, which felt like an eternity to me, my son again rounded that corner, but toward me, and he was beaming. I will never forget that look of pride on his face. We had both made it through.

I have a few favorite ways to use lists for my own family, and my clients love them too. Here are a few examples:

Morning responsibilities

I mentioned before that one of my sons has a hard time remembering what he needs to do in the morning to get out the door. We have a list on the fridge with all of his responsibilities including:

- Brush teeth
- Pack lunch and snack in backpack
- Put shoes on
- Kiss dogs goodbye
- Hug Mom and Dad

I don't have to nag him about the same things day in and day out because after he eats I can simply remind him to look at his list.

Grocery lists

One of my private coaching clients was having a hard time running her household because she felt like her husband and kids were telling her things they needed in passing, and she would forget to write them down because she was usually in the middle of something else. We devised a system where she had a whiteboard in her office for a list of items that her husband and teenage kids needed. The list included things like shaving cream, deodorant, school supplies, and various other things. She told them that she would buy anything that was on the list for them when she went to the store, but there was to be no more mentioning items in passing. If it was on the list, it would be bought, but if not, tough luck.

Once everyone got a bit of practice remembering to write things on the list, the flow of errands was much easier because she could get all the requested items in one trip instead of running around like a crazy person every time there was a new request. Her husband and kids knew that she would purchase the items on her next shopping trip.

You could also keep a list on the fridge or the kitchen counter. It doesn't matter where, as long as it gets used!

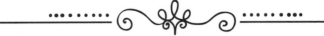

Weekly schedules

I sometimes feel like my kids have way more going on in their lives than I do! Between sports and birthday parties, they are kept very busy. Sometimes *too* busy!

Different days require different equipment, whether it be for soccer, baseball, basketball, gymnastics, ballet, or tutoring. It can be hard to keep it all straight, and that's where having a list can be really helpful.

I like using a whiteboard in a central location like the kitchen or mudroom that lists out which kids have what activity on a given day and then what equipment is needed for that activity. For example, if they were going to soccer, they would need a water bottle, cleats, their uniform, and a ball. If they were going to tutoring, they need the books and folders required for that session. Having a list with everything that needs to be packed makes it easier to walk out the door and minimizes the times you have to run back home because you forgot something.

Kids can look at these lists and help get organized, and it can even be done the night before so there is one less thing to do in the morning or after school.

Evening responsibilities

When my kids were little, bath time was a huge part of our routine. Evenings that I was exhausted, bath time would stretch into a full-on activity because the kids were happy and contained, and I just got to sit next to the tub and kvell over how adorable they were pouring water over each other's heads.

As the kids got a bit older and evenings began to consist of shuttling to sports practices and Hebrew school, bathtime turned into

shower time and often became something that took just a few minutes. Kids can help prepare for bedtime and the next day by being in charge of brushing teeth, laying out clothes for school the next day, or girlie things that I know my nieces need to do, like cleaning their earring holes with alcohol each night for a few weeks after they got their ears pierced. If there are more than two or three items that you want kids to remember, I would make a list for the bathroom mirror or inside their closet for sure.

Gift lists

Gift lists are one of the best things that ever happened to parents! Both of my boys have birthdays in early summer, about halfway through the year from the Christmas/Hanukkah season. This means that I have roughly six months that my kids can make a Hanukkah list, and about six months that they can make a birthday list.

Every time my kids ask me for something random that they don't need, I tell them to add it to their gift list so when people ask what they want for Hanukkah or their birthday I will be armed and ready with the information.

Gold star lists/compliments

Some lists are just about feeling good, and that is important, too! Think about how amazing it feels to receive a heartfelt compliment. Really, really good, right? Well, kids think so, too!

Wouldn't it be nice to keep a running list all week of what your kids do that really stands out as being kind or exemplary in some way, and then once a week or once a month you can read that list at dinner? Just imagine the beams of pride radiating off them when you

do. Let's encourage them to do more by celebrating these acts and letting them know that we truly notice and appreciate them.

Chore lists

We've mentioned ways to divvy up chores, but keeping track can be helpful too. If your kids are responsible for chores in your home, help them keep a list of what they are so they have a way to keep track of what has been done.

There are many schools of thought on whether chores should be done simply because you are a member of a household and you need to help or for an allowance. There isn't one right way to think about this, and each family should do what they are comfortable with. I do, however, like the idea of celebrating a completed chore list as a family by doing something fun together. Maybe it's simply sharing a Popsicle or ice cream in the backyard, playing a game, or all grabbing a book and just vegging together for thirty minutes. It's about working hard together and playing hard together!

Sleepover lists

One great place to foster independence is getting ready for sleepovers. For the first few years that my kids were sleeping out, I packed and unpacked their bag for them. It dawned on me one day that my kids wouldn't have any experience packing or unpacking if I never let them do it. For a while we packed their bags together, and then one day I gave them the task of getting all of their stuff together and they did great.

It would be helpful if you or your kids are nervous about forgetting items to make a sleepover list and either keep it taped to the

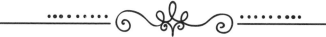

inside of their closet or even in a designated sleepover bag. This way a toothbrush always makes it into the bag!

Instead of my kids coming home the next morning and dumping their bag for me to deal with, they now have to take it up and unpack it, including putting the laundry in the laundry room. Next up needs to be actually doing the laundry!

27

Get Your Kids to THINK

Kiss name-calling goodbye

"Raise your words, not your voice. It's rain that grows flowers, not thunder."
—RUMI

A colleague of mine, Cynthia Kane, wrote a book filled with wisdom. It's called *How to Communicate Like a Buddhist.* In it, she teaches the elements of right speech (speech that avoids harming and lacks ill will) that stem from Buddhist teaching in a way that feels applicable and relatable to our modern, everyday lives. The four right parts of speech are: 1. Tell the truth, 2. Don't exaggerate, 3. Don't gossip, and 4. Use helpful language. If you were considering these guidelines for your communication with others and with yourself, what would you need to change? It can be a scary question when we begin to truly examine how we speak.

Modeling conscious language can feel difficult as a parent because we may not have really concentrated on it before, but it is our duty to teach our children how to speak and react with kindness and mindfulness.

We were having issues with name-calling in my home, and I knew that I needed to get the situation under control quickly before my younger son had permanent damage to his self-esteem and psyche thanks to unkind words he was hearing from his older brother. Every single time he opened his mouth to say anything, he heard something along the lines of, "You are so stupid" from his brother whom he not only loved, but downright worshiped. Obviously this was not okay, but no matter how many times my husband and I spoke to our older son about it, it didn't subside. It almost became like a knee-jerk reaction. I wondered if he had developed some kind of tic or automatic response to his brother's voice, and it broke my heart on both counts. I was sad for my little one to hear such unkind words day in and day out, and I was sad that my older son had it in him to make someone feel so bad. As sweet and loving as he usually is, this was not kind or acceptable and I couldn't let it continue.

I knew I needed to get to my older son in a different way since our talks weren't working, so I printed out a sign and posted it on our fridge that said:

Before you speak you need to THINK!

T—is it true?

H—is it helpful?

I—is it inspiring?

N—is it necessary?

K—is it kind?

I sat down with the two boys, and we began to discuss what these questions meant. How before we speak, we need to THINK and ask ourselves these questions. If the answer to any of them is "no," then maybe we should think twice before saying something.

We ran through some examples. I would say something and they would have to determine if I had used this criteria. Then they took

turns practicing, and over time it helped to create a new language in our household. If Adam said something unkind to Dylan, he didn't hear the same old, tired speech of, "That wasn't nice. What made you say that? You need to say sorry," which usually went in one ear and out the other and tended to evoke an un-heartfelt apology that didn't make anyone feel better.

But now I had a whole new script ready, and when we change things up, kids notice. If something unkind was said, I began to ask if he used THINK before he spoke, and then we would break down the parts, and I would ask if what he said was true, helpful, inspiring, necessary, or kind. Once he was forced to answer questions like, "Is your brother really stupid? I mean do you really, honestly, and truly think he is stupid? Is it helpful to tell him he is stupid? Do you think that inspires him?" he began to get it. And he stopped.

Mom. Win.

I love this strategy because it just plain makes sense to kids. It gives a common language to use that everyone understands, and it gave me a way to talk to my kids that didn't lead to yelling even when I was boiling and sad on the inside. I basically had a script that got to my kids on a different level. It didn't go in one ear and out the other. After answering these questions Adam truly did feel sorry. He understood how hurtful his words were, and he apologized from a heartfelt place instead of because he was forced to.

These questions also made me consider my own right speech. There were times that I admittedly said things in judgment of another, or myself, and the answers to these questions was undoubtedly "no." These questions have helped me to be more mindful about what is coming out of my own mouth, ultimately making me a better role model for my kids and those around me.

One of the five essentials of meditation that I discussed in chapter 14 is be kind to yourself. Are you? Really? I love how Cynthia describes that: "The words we speak to ourselves over and over become our beliefs, and if we are feeding ourselves a diet of negative self-talk, we create an environment of suffering. If we start speaking to ourselves in a kind, honest, nonjudgmental, and helpful way, then we are far more likely to create interactions with others that follow these same rules." Yup.

Cynthia and I agree on something very major. We cannot control what others do, but we can control what we do. If someone is gossiping, we cannot control that, but we can control whether or not we participate and engage. Also, if you find that you are berating yourself internally, you have a choice of continuing or catching yourself in the act and working to break the habit.

I simply adore the work of the author, speaker, and spiritual teacher Byron Katie, and it pops into my mind every time I am having an unkind thought whether it is about myself or someone else. I ask myself, "Is that thought true? Is there a stress-free reason to keep that thought?" and the most life-changing one for me, "Who would I be without that thought?" The answer is usually happier, more content, and more centered.

All of these questions are basically retraining our brain to eventually think differently. As I write this I am currently experiencing a "brain retrain" myself—I am participating in a twenty-one-day consecutive no-complaining challenge, based on the concepts taught in Will Bowen's book *A Complaint Free World*. I have to say that it is harder than I thought!

I was invited to a seminar on the challenge by my friend who said, "This is so up your alley," and she was spot-on. Even though I don't think of myself as a huge complainer, I am always looking

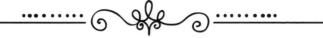

to grow and improve myself. I wasn't sure if I would be able to go because one of my kids had a game at that time, but something happened and it got moved, so I felt like the Universe was opening up the space for me to attend. How could I say "no" to that?

The point of the challenge is to not complain for twenty-one days *in a row*. So no matter what day you are on, if you complain, you have to start over. Our facilitator explained that it typically takes individuals four to six months to complete the challenge. At the time of writing this I have been doing the challenge for five weeks, and I have had to start over eleven times. Honestly, I am really surprised by this! I had expectations of flying through the challenge and beating all my friends. I definitely have more work to do than I thought.

Complaining is a low-vibe behavior and is a really unhealthy way to try to connect with other people. But I can tell you firsthand that it takes awareness, patience, and commitment to change, just as the group leader teaching us said it would. It was also brought to our attention that the average person complains fifteen to thirty times a day. That is a *lot* of complaining!

During the 21-Day Challenge, you wear a wristband that says "complain free world" on it, and every time you complain you switch what wrist it is on.

A big part of the challenge is figuring out what is actually a complaint and what is a statement. For example, if you stub your toe and it hurts, you can certainly say "Ow!" That is not a complaint. If you go on to say that "That effing hurt and this is the worst day ever and how come the world is against me and nothing good ever happens to me," then you definitely need to start over! It is much more about the intention behind your statements.

I decided to bring the principle I teach of using your body to help you make decisions into the challenge to help me determine

if something is a complaint. Remember when I taught you about the "yums" and the "yucks?" Well, they became my rule of thumb so I knew when I needed to start over. If I said something and I got a "yuck" feeling in the pit of my stomach or felt regret at saying it, that was my body's signal that it was a complaint. I basically used my body instead of my mind, because my body doesn't get confused. This really helped me, and I shared it with a few friends doing the challenge, and they used this as a gauge as well.

There are four stages to the challenge:

- Unconscious Incompetent is when you are not aware of your complaining.
- Conscious Incompetent is when you are aware of complaining, but you can't stop. This is the stage where you are constantly starting over.
- Conscious Competent is when you are aware and you don't want to switch your wristband so you catch yourself. Even though you may think something in your head, you don't let it come out of your mouth.
- Unconscious Competence is when you don't have to think about not complaining anymore. You have truly solidified your new habit of not complaining because your thoughts have actually changed.

It is amazing how completely obvious what stage you are in is. I am currently still in stage two. It is time to get serious and move to stage three! I don't know how long my brain retrain will take, but I have gained so much more awareness, and as we know, that is the key to change.

During the challenge you are supposed to congratulate yourself on your awareness with a phrase like, "Congratulations, I caught a

behavior that I want to change. I am aware of myself." This a huge step because the book states that "Complaining is like bad breath. You notice it on other people." But after this challenge I have gained the awareness needed to correct my own behavior.

This challenge has taught me a few things indeed, such as:

- I complain more than I thought.
- Everyone is on their own journey, and instead of thinking of others as "complainers," I now just see them as being in a different stage than me.
- It is hard to do a brain retrain! This gives me a bit more compassion for my kids when I am trying to help them retrain their brains and it takes a bit longer than I am expecting.

When we stop complaining we are better able to address issues head on. Another thing that I like about the challenge is that it is extremely realistic. Sometimes you need to discuss an issue going on in your life with someone. If you are doing it simply to vent and bitch, without wanting to find a solution or a way to move forward, that is complaining. But if you want to open up about your feelings to a close friend or loved one in the hopes that they can help you sort through your feelings and find the best way to proceed in a positive direction, then that is not complaining. Again, it's all about the intention behind your words. Complaining keeps us focused on the problem instead of moving toward a solution. But now we can move forward instead of staying stuck in negativity.

I love the way the following concept was explained in the workshop. Our brain is the manufacturer, and our mouth is the consumer. When there is no longer a demand for complaints, our brain will stop producing them.

By the time this book is in your hands, I fully expect to be finished and enjoying stage four, no longer manufacturing complaints.

Would you ever consider doing your own challenge?

Section 3

Mindful Mom Moments

We can be so busy teaching our kids about respect, boundaries, and important life lessons, that we forget to just enjoy them! They are only young once. We need to be present and take advantage of every opportunity that we have to bond and connect.

The following lessons are comprised of ideas for creating true connection with our kiddos, and inviting them to feel valued and heard. Take the time to create memories that will stand out as fun and meaningful when they are adults.

A few years ago, I wrote my mom a letter and listed all the great memories I had from childhood that she was a part of. It was a compilation of small moments like how I used to lay with my head in her lap and she would tickle my back on long drives (before the days of seatbelts!). I mentioned how she could whip up a yummy dinner when I thought the fridge looked bare, how she always called fruit "luscious," and how she used to come talk about art to my class growing up.

There wasn't one thing I remembered that was a "thing." Not one instance was about anything she ever bought for me. It was all

about the times we spent together doing the little things. I can only hope and pray that I am creating the same lasting memories for my own kids. When they look back on their childhood, I want them to remember that we played games and laughed together, that I taught them to breathe easy, and that I snuggled with them every night before bed.

I hope you gain a bit of inspiration from the next few chapters. My goal is to give you at least one new idea that you read about and think, "We are totally doing this today!"

Promise me you won't wait to bond, because we don't find the time for what is important to us, we *make* the time.

28

Quantity over Quality

We've all heard it, but let's do it!

"While we try to teach our children all about life, our children teach us what life is all about."

—ANGELA SCHWINDT

Have you ever had a super fun day with the kiddos where you really felt connected, but if someone asked you what you did you'd answer, "Nothing much?" Those are some of my favorite days! Don't get me wrong, I absolutely love traveling with my children and creating beautiful memories by experiencing something new together. We also have exciting days made up of professional sporting events, occasional Broadway shows while visiting family in New York, and more mainstream activities like bowling, movies, and arcades. They are fun for sure, but sometimes sitting around the kitchen table over sandwiches or snuggling in bed at night is when I feel like the real bonding happens. I hope they are soaking up and savoring the little things that bind our family together. I know I am.

When I spoke about meditation I mentioned quantity over quality. Let me take a moment to remind you that how often we meditate is more important than how we view the quality of our meditations. They are all good! I think that phrase is perfectly applicable when we talk about bonding with our kids and the time we spend with them as well. Kids need us. They need lots of us. They need to know that we enjoy spending time with them, and it honestly doesn't matter what we are doing as long as we are together. It is quantity over quality. Running errands can be fun if you are together! Every time we are with our kids it isn't about a big, fancy, planned date or buying something. I believe that it really takes time and energy to form close bonds, and as fun as special outings are, there are a few low-key ways that I love to really connect with my kids. Here are a few of my faves:

Making eye contact

Sure, we talk to our kids, but are you really looking at each other when you do? Eye contact solidifies connection. It lets someone know that you are really listening to them. Take one day and pay attention to how many times you are looking at your kids when you talk to them. It may surprise you.

Aim for making eye contact a minimum of five times per day. Yelling from the kitchen to get shoes on doesn't count!

When we help our children practice making eye contact, we are also helping them develop a life skill. They get to practice with us in a safe environment so it's easier when they are talking to teachers, relatives, and friends' parents. The ability to maintain eye contact shows someone that you are truly listening and paying attention. It shows respect and builds trust.

A study done by www.studybodylanguage.com implied that people who maintain eye contact are perceived as reliable, warm, sociable, honest, and confident. Many children don't feel comfortable making eye contact with adults, so allowing them to practice at home with us can be extremely beneficial.

Sharing stories about my childhood

My kids *love* to hear stories about my childhood. It's fun to share that my twin sister and I had our own language that nobody else could understand. I've shared with my little one that my older sister used to make me sit at her door when her friends were over. I could never actually come in, and I didn't care. I just wanted to be near her! I've told them about learning to scuba dive as a teenager and that I went on a dive with sharks, which may be one of the most daring things I have ever done. They stared at me wide-eyed when they learned why I had three fake teeth—I fell off a horse at camp when I was fourteen and was dragged for a hundred yards on my face. Ouch! My boys soak it up when I explain to them that all my birthday parties when I was young were at home and we played games like Duck, Duck, Goose, and my mom made my twin sister and I an ice cream cake every year. They can't believe that I used to break up with my twin sister's boyfriends on the phone and she used to quit my jobs because our voices are identical. They giggle when they hear that I used to tell people that I had a brother named Homer, who was really our dog.

Share with your kids! Fiction is fun, but you can't beat reality, and it helps our kids to know us, just as it helps us bond with them. Not to mention, it's really fun to remember things that you haven't thought of in years!

Finding times that I can say "Yes!"

I remember one day when I was standing at the kitchen sink with gloves on, making my way through a pile of dishes. I was up to my elbows in hot, soapy water scrubbing a pot when my son walked over and asked me to play a game.

My first inclination was to tell him that I would after I was done doing the dishes, but then I thought to myself, *Does it really matter if I play first or do dishes first?* So I took off my gloves and told him to pick out a game. His eyes were bright and wide, and I could tell how much it meant to him that I said "Yes" and didn't put him off. He won against the dishes!

We can't always do this because some timelines do matter, like putting younger siblings to bed or having a scheduled appointment. But there are times when it truly doesn't matter and something can wait. Take advantage of them. Find times to say "Yes!" I'm not sure who will feel better about it—you or your kids.

I manage a Facebook group called "Hot Mess to Mindful Mom Community," full of women that inspire and support each other to live their best lives as moms and women. We share wins, challenges, and ideas so we feel less alone on this journey to mindful parenting. If you are looking to join an active community of moms with a relatable, authentic, and low-key vibe, check it out on Facebook!

When I was writing this chapter, I decided to poll the moms in the *Hot Mess to Mindful Mom* Community group to see what their favorite ways to bond with their kids were. I got some great answers and ideas! Here are a few:

- Wrestling
- Funny staring games

- Hand games
- Family outings
- Board games
- Coloring
- Letting the kids guide through a museum (love that!)
- Hiking
- Baking
- Telling embarrassing stories
- Telling scary stories
- Family yoga
- Painting
- Dance parties (the best!)
- Watch movies
- Play basketball
- Juicing
- Cooking
- Reading (a staple)

This just goes to show that there is no wrong way to bond with your kiddos, and anything goes as long as you are enjoying time with each other.

29

Copy Your Kids

Live in the moment

"It's not only children who grow. Parents do too. As much as we watch to see what our children do with their lives, they are watching to see what we do with ours."
—Joyce Maynard

When I began to collect ideas related to living in the moment I immediately thought of video games. My kids are not huge gamers, but I know tons of kids that are really into them. That isn't to say that my older son couldn't make music videos on his phone for hours on end and my little one wouldn't be happy watching Netflix all the live-long day. They like technology just fine, thank you, but we don't have traditional video games like Playstation and Xbox at our house anymore.

I started doing a bit of research on video games and I came across an article on the website Raise Smart Kid that surprised me. It was about the positive and negative effects of video games, and the part that was shocking was that both arguments were equally as long. I

didn't know there actually were that many good things about video games. A few that stood out were:

- They can help kids learn to follow instructions.
- They can help increase problem-solving and logic.
- They can improve hand-eye coordination, fine motor, and spatial skills.
- They can help develop reading and math skills.
- They can help develop perseverance.
- They can help increase pattern recognition.
- They can help with mapping skills.
- They can help improve how kids respond to frustration and rethinking goals.
- They can make learning fun.
- They can help parents and kids play together.
- They can help improve eyesight.
- They can help kids with dyslexia read faster and with more accuracy.

And then I got to the part of the article that talked about the negative effects of video games, such as:

- Violent video games can lead to more aggressive thoughts, feelings, and behaviors, and decreased prosocial helping.
- There is a consistent correlation between violent game use and aggression.
- They can make kids socially isolated and may lead to less time spent on homework, reading, sports, and interacting with friends and family.
- Games can confuse fantasy and reality.

- The more time a kid spends playing video games, the poorer his or her performance is in school.
- Overuse can lead to obesity, nerve compression, and carpal tunnel syndrome.
- Games can be addictive, and this addictive behavior can lead to increased depression and anxiety.

To be honest, from my mom perspective, violent video games have always freaked me out, but I do understand that we need to read this data and understand it for what it is. For video games to have a positive influence, it sounds like they would need to be educational for starters. I am not sure how realistic that is 100 percent of the time.

On the flip side, the negative effects seem to come mostly from violent games, and playing video games for extended periods of time every day.

Our job as parents is to monitor video and screen time, notice the effects they have on our children, vary the choices that our kids have for entertainment, and be sure that they are getting enough physical activity. If we see a drop in grades or an increase in aggression, we may need to rethink the time they are spending gaming.

The reason I brought up video games to begin with is because I have always been amazed at the level of concentration that kids have when they are playing these games. It intrigues me. The ability to mono-task is something that many adults can learn from, myself included. I am always striving to improve in this area.

For years we have heard how great multi-tasking is, but there is a swing in the pendulum moving us toward mono-tasking. This is because when you multi-task you get less done and you do it poorly. It is easy to get distracted, especially when it comes to social media and technology. When you mono-task you actually get more done and you do it better because you actually finish what you start, and

are truly engaged and focused on your task. I love how fastcompany. com stated that "mono-tasking is the new multi-tasking."

How can we train our kids, and ourselves for that matter, to use the same level of concentration they use while playing video games when they are doing other meaningful activities like homework or socializing? Here are a few ideas:

Build up your stamina

Everyone has a different tolerance for mono-tasking, and it's important to know what that is. Mine is about an hour. I tell myself that if I write for an hour I can check my e-mail or make tea when I am done. If I try to force myself to go longer than an hour, I feel extremely distracted. It works really well for adults and kids to use a timer. For example, kids can do homework for twenty minutes (or whatever their tolerance is), and when their timer goes off they can get a drink, go to the bathroom, or play a quick game of cards with you, and then it's back to hitting the books.

Limit distractions

If you grab your phone every two seconds to check Instagram when you should be working, or even while watching television or reading, move it! Remember, we are striving to do one thing at a time. I have to do this myself.

Be compassionate toward yourself

We cannot expect our habits and behaviors to change overnight. It's not like you're going to give yourself a little pep talk and then its

mono-tasking from here on out. This is a new skill that we must practice. The goal is to gain awareness, and to get better over time.

Practice saying "No" nicely

I have talked about this before, but it really applies here as well. You will occasionally need to say no to something that interferes with mono-tasking. It took me a while to grasp the concept that I didn't have to answer the phone every single time it rang. If I am in the middle of something and it isn't school or my husband calling, then it can wait. If I am working on a big project, like a book, I have to say no to other things because I won't be successful if my attention is divided in so many directions. Sometimes I have to choose me and my work, and that is okay!

When our kids are playing or riding bikes or reading, they are fully engaged in their activity. It is amazing as parents to give our kids that same undivided attention that they so crave from us. I have seen relationships that my clients have with their kids change when they are giving them positive, undivided attention. Their kids don't have to go looking to get their attention in other ways like acting out.

There are so many ways to give our kids undivided attention, and it doesn't have to be for an entire afternoon to be meaningful. Short spurts accomplish just as much, and this should be a low-pressure activity. Special dates don't have to be elaborate plans or expensive in any way. Time is the currency here.

One great way to start is to set a timer for twenty or thirty minutes and let your child direct the play at home. You don't even have to leave the house to bond and connect! Put your phone far away so you won't be distracted (or at least turn off the notifications). If your mind wanders, come back to your child's eyes, their giggle, and

whatever the game is at hand. They will be so happy to have your undivided attention and you will feel like parent of the year!

One of my clients has three children and was worried about giving equal special time to each of them. I encouraged her to put a chart on the fridge, and she marked off when she had a special little date with each child each week. Time can easily get away from us, so this tool proved very helpful for keeping track, and it motivated her to stay on top of their dates.

One of my favorite things to do is to take my kids to Starbucks for a hot chocolate along with a deck of cards We play Gin or Spit as we talk and share. It is easy, inexpensive, and always fun.

Cooking or baking together is always a great option, as is reading, painting nails, or playing catch. There is absolutely no way to mess this up as long as you are spending time together and enjoying each other.

Imagine how your relationship with your kids will thrive if you are really present in the moment with them on a regular basis. Think about the skills that you can help them develop as well.

In this day and age kids spend more time with their heads turned toward a screen than actual people, and I keep hearing about the epidemic that teens and young adults don't have the same communication skills we did growing up. We need to give them a chance to practice. How do we do that? It isn't by half-listening while we scroll through Facebook ourselves! We need to communicate with our kids by talking to them, looking them in the eye, and modeling for them how to really pay attention. If we don't, how will they see what this looks like in action?

Presence is power. We want our kids to grow up to be contributing members of society, to have a voice in the workplace, and to be interesting conversationalists. We want our kids to learn to speak

confidently, manage social situations with ease and grace, and to follow their intuition. Just like any other skills in life, these don't come
out of the blue. They must be nurtured and developed.

These moments of true presence are also a chance for us to pause
in our busy day, settle our nervous system, and bring more joy into
our life. Let's face it, we probably need to practice these skills as
much as our kids!

30

Family Rituals

Make memories your kids will never forget!

*"Listen earnestly to anything your children want to tell you no matter what. If you
don't listen eagerly to the little stuff when they are little, they won't tell you the big
stuff when they are big, because to them all of it has always been big stuff."*

—CATHERINE WALLACE

Things were *so* different when I was growing up. I vividly remember
a time when my twin sister and I were about eight years old. We
were in the backseat of my dad's car, and we were fighting like cats
and dogs. I don't remember why now, but we must have been in
full-on brat mode. My dad repeatedly told us to stop, but of course
we didn't. Eventually he threatened to kick us out of the car. We
continued to fight, so he made good on his word and pulled the car
over and made us get out. My sister and I stood on the corner staring
at each other as my dad drove away. He must have circled the block a
few times and come right back, but of course it felt like forever to us.
When he pulled back up we silently got into the car and were quiet

all the way home. In today's day and age I would be scared about someone calling CPS if I tried that move!

One of my happiest memories is how we used to ride our bikes for hours after school and on the weekends, and my parents had no clue where we were. They felt totally safe with this arrangement and so did we. I can't even imagine that today. If my son walks to his friend's around the corner he calls me from his phone to let me know that he arrived. It's a different world. It makes me a bit sad that my kids will never know that kind of freedom.

I am one of four girls, and when one of us was sick growing up, the rest of us would fake sick so that we could spend the entire day together watching TV. We would make our schedule by circling the TV Guide, and even though we only had three channels because we didn't have cable, it was still so fun. We would call the drugstore that delivered as we watched "Price is Right," and order Luden's cherry and lemon cough drops and gum. We took turns getting up to turn the dial on the small television set to change channels. Those were days I will never forget.

Our most important ritual growing up was Candy Night. We were not allowed to have junk food during the week, as my mom was ahead of her time on the health food front, but once a week on Saturday night we were allowed to have one candy bar. We went to the drugstore each Saturday afternoon and debated which one would last the longest. I remember Charleston Chew being a very popular choice. A Charleston Chew could last all the way through *The Muppet Show* and *The Barbara Mandrel Show.* Maybe even through *The Love Boat*!

I am sure my parents didn't devise Candy Night anticipating that it would be one of my most vivid childhood memories, but it is, which goes to show that we don't know what will stick with our own

kids. I want my boys to have fond memories and experiences that define their childhood in the very same way.

The most popular ritual in our home is birthday room decorating. Ever since my kids turned two, we have decorated their room in a different way every single birthday. From balloon drops over their bed to streamers covering it, Mark and I have exhausted every option at the party supply store. We fret for weeks before their birthday that we won't be able to think of something new, but we haven't failed yet! The kids speculate for weeks and truly look forward to seeing what we are going to do, which makes it worth the pressure. This is something they will tell their own kids about.

Just like special dates, rituals don't have to be grand or expensive gestures. It's the repetition of them, and the idea behind them that makes them special. Whether they take place once a year, or once a week, I encourage you to create some sort of family ritual. Here are a few ideas to get you started:

- Weekly or monthly "dates" from the previous chapter
- Coloring together (I love mindful coloring, and if you haven't jumped on the bandwagon yet, give it a go!)
- Family game nights
- Breakfast in bed on birthdays
- Dessert for breakfast on birthdays
- Holiday baking
- Making and delivering treats for neighbors during the holidays
- Sunday night movie night
- Weekly family meetings
- Volunteering together (once a month or during the holidays)
- Family bike rides
- Family workouts

- Working on large puzzles together
- Yearly trips to a favorite vacation spot
- Girlie spa days together
- Watching a favorite sport together on television
- Parent/child book club
- Having a shared journal and writing notes back and forth
- Friday night "The Weekend's Here!" dance parties
- Bring your child to work days
- Family picnics/indoor picnics

If something feels really fun as a family, mark your calendar to do it once a week, once a month, or every so often. Give yourself reminders when life feels busy. It's totally worth it!

By taking the time to create and nurture these rituals, we have the opportunity to bring an even deeper meaning to them. A client I spoke to recently about these types of family rituals said that they were completely missing from her life growing up. She told me that if something like this had been a part of her childhood, she would have felt more secure and confident.

Rituals help kids to feel supported and add stability to their lives. They can also be comforting to us as adults. Do you have rituals in your own life? Do you go to the same coffee shop on the way to work? Do you order Chinese food on Sunday nights? Do you make the same smoothie after your workouts? Do you call your husband or best friend from the car each day? How do these rituals make you feel? Most likely safe, secure, and loved. If it feels this good to us, let's be sure we are giving this to our kids.

31

Dream Together

Have a vision board party!

"The future belongs to those who believe in the beauty of their dreams."
—ELEANOR ROOSEVELT

I remember vividly the night that Gabby Bernstein announced she was doing her very first Spirit Junkie Master Class in New York City. I was on her webinar when it was announced, and I knew with every ounce of my being that I belonged in that audience.

I took my husband up to my altar which was then in my closet, and I asked him, "What do you notice when you look at all this stuff?" He looked around and said, "You really like that girl," pointing to the beautiful blonde on my vision board. I answered, "That's right. And I'm going to meet her. I am going to New York City to meet her."

Meeting Gabby was on my vision board, and I did meet her that year. Sarah McLean was on my board, and I have now studied under her and I consider her a dear friend. There was a beautiful beach

amongst the pictures, and I have visited a few of those since I made my board as well. Oprah and a picture of India were also on there, but I tell the Universe that I can be patient. I am holding the vision!

Have you ever made a vision board?

Visualization is another great way to manifest, and a vision board is an extremely valuable tool that represents your dreams, goals, and how you want to feel in your life.

According to an article by Jack Canfield, "Because your mind responds strongly to visual stimulation, by representing your goals with pictures and images, you actually strengthen and stimulate your emotions . . . and your emotions are the vibrational energy that activates the Law of Attraction." This is why the saying "A picture is worth a thousand words" is so true!

Christine Kane also explains that, "The idea behind vision boards is that when you surround yourself with images of who you want to become, what you want to have, where you want to live, or where you want to vacation, your life changes to match those images and desires."

I started laughing while I was doing research on this topic when I came across an article in the *Huffington Post* that stated, "If you think vision boards are bogus, then the joke's on you." The article goes on to explain that creating a sacred space that displays what you want actually does bring it to life. What we focus on expands, and when looking at your vision board throughout the day, you are constantly doing short visualization exercises.

The book *The Secret* purports that when we visualize, we emit a powerful frequency out into the Universe, which is the Law of Attraction. This is why Olympic athletes have been using visualization to improve performance for years. That and taking huge amounts of inspired action, of course. Olympic athletes don't sit on their couch

dreaming of gold. They are up and at 'em day in and day out, busting their tushies off. That hard work, along with seeing their dreams come true in their mind, and feeling it in their gut, is how the magic happens.

The secret, according the *Huffington Post*, is that your vision board should focus on how you want to feel, not just on the things that you want. Of course you can and should also include material things if you want, but the more your board focuses on how you want to feel, the more it will come to life.

If someone makes a vision board and feels like nothing is happening, this could be the missing piece. It is easy to say that we want something in our life, whether it be clients or new clothes, but we need to take it another step and get to the root of the feelings behind it. Helping that client makes you feel empowered, loving, and helpful. New clothes make you feel confident, pulled together, and beautiful.

Now that we have covered that vision boards can really help bring our goals to fruition, how do we go about making one?

A vision board can encompass goals and dreams in all areas of your life, or you can make one that is more specific, for example one that concentrates on work goals.

I encourage you to sit quietly in meditation, or just in a quiet state, and really let your heart speak. Get in touch with your highest self and focus on what you are hoping to bring into your life. Set your visions and intentions.

Get a poster board or cork board. Find pictures, quotes, affirmations, or inspiring words that represent your goals and desires. You can find them in magazines, on the Internet, or you can write some of your own. You can also attach meaningful mementos that conjure up feelings for you, such as a brochure or a napkin from somewhere

that you want to visit, or visit again. You can use photographs or even draw some of your own pictures. Consider putting a picture of yourself on your board.

Before you glue with rubber cement or a glue stick, lay out all the pictures and quotes and various other things that you pulled for your board. Listen to your intuition and lay your favorites on your board. Remove anything that no longer calls to you. Organize the images in a way that feels natural to you. Do you like them separated into themes or are you drawn to a more fluid layout?

Your board should reflect your personality and your dream life. If you don't like clutter around you in your day to day life, keep your board nice and neat and not overstuffed.

Each year you can "clean up" your board. If something has come to fruition, take a moment to acknowledge that and be grateful for it. You don't necessarily have to remove it because it is a great visual reminder that you deliberately attracted and manifested something into your life. However, maybe some goals have shifted for you in some way and you need to change some words or pictures out.

Jack Canfield had a few tips (quoted below) for utilizing your vision board on his website, and I thought they were great:

- Look at your vision board often and feel the inspiration it provides.
- Hold it in your hands and really internalize the future it represents.
- Read your affirmations and inspirational words aloud.
- See yourself living in that manner.
- Feel yourself in the future you have designed.
- Believe it is already yours.
- Be grateful for the good that is already present in your life.

- Acknowledge any goals you have already achieved.
- Acknowledge the changes you have seen and felt.
- Look at it just before going to bed and first thing in the morning.

If you don't know *exactly* what you want to call into your life, you can still make a vision board. Make it about how you want to feel. Pull pictures and quotes that make you feel good and don't even think about why while you pull. Stay open-minded and simply let your intuition speak. You may even learn about some of your heartfelt desires that you never realized were there.

Like everything I have learned along my spiritual and self-care journey, it would have been amazing to know it *sooner*! I know we can't look back, and everything comes to us in divine timing, but I can't help but wonder what mistakes and stressors I could have avoided had I begun meditating ten years earlier!

Wouldn't it be great if we could introduce our children to vision boarding? Why not make it a family affair!

Get creative with your kids and guide them as they set goals and intentions. Make an afternoon of it with fun music and a brainstorming session. Kids may need a bit of guidance to get going, but we have the incredible opportunity to model dreaming big for them. Once they see you start they will get the idea!

Use this as an opportunity to encourage your kids to dream big. Where do they want to travel one day? How do they want to feel in school? What activities do they want to try? What instruments do they want to play? I bet you will find out some amazing things about your kids that you didn't already know, and they will learn about you as well.

Bust out magazines and markers, photo albums and paint, and let your kids have a ball getting creative with their dreams. I bet you will learn a ton about them in the process.

A few more tips that I picked up from "The Mama Mary Show" to make vision boarding kid-friendly are:

- Make sure your magazines are kid-friendly. Pop culture and cooking mags are okay, but throw in some Disney or *Sports Illustrated Kids* and the like, too.
- Explain how the night will work; set expectations and time limits. Create an overall plan and discuss how much time you are allotting to each part of the project. Some time will be spent looking for pictures in magazines and online, some time to cutting and gluing, and time at the end to present their board.
- Consider calling them dream boards instead of vision boards. It's just more kid-friendly language!
- Know where they will be displayed.

If they are too big it may be hard to have a spot. Smaller, thinner boards may be easier to tape on a wall in their room.

Making a vision board can help Type-A, super-logical kids embrace their creativity and create a safe forum to simply dream without wondering about the how's and why's. They can tap into their intuition and desires without the fear of being judged by others or themselves. They can take themselves out of the box and release any self-inflicted or societal limits. Think total freedom to dream.

Creating a board and choosing images and words can also help kids uncover their own limiting beliefs with you as their guide. If they start to pull a picture and then hesitate because they think they can't have something, maybe it's time for a heart-to-heart conversation with them. Create a safe space for them to open up about their feelings.

As adults we have many stories that we created in our heads over years and years. If we bombed a math test as a kid, we may have created a story that we aren't good in math, and are attached to that thought. That thought and belief may have even dictated a career choice, or whether we think we can tackle certain projects. Who would we be without that thought?

It's funny because I grew up believing that I was terrible at sports. I became attached to that thought early on in life, and therefore never really tried or put much effort in because I didn't think it was worth it. It wasn't until I was an adult that I realized that I am a great runner; in fact, when I was thirty-six, I ran my first marathon.

I also realized on a family vacation at thirty-nine that I am a kick-ass wake boarder! I decided to try, really to impress my kids, and I got right up and was the best on the boat. It was exhilarating to see myself be good after spending so long thinking that I suck at anything athletic. That will go down as one of my proudest moments because of how it made me feel inside.

Wouldn't it be wonderful if we could help our kids detach from the types of thoughts that eventually turn into limiting beliefs? We can help them shift their blocks and live their full potential, but only if we can get them to open up about how they are feeling. Creating a fun and engaging atmosphere, like making a vision board together, can allow them to feel safe and comfortable enough to let out their fears and feelings. This is as in-the-moment as we can get. I am not sure a conversation like this would ordinarily present itself without a child feeling insecure or defensive.

32

How to Have Time for You without Dissing Your Family

We all need down time

"You know you're a mom when all you want is some time alone, but you miss the kids as soon as you get it."

—MOMMY WISE

I have had people say some crazy things to me over the years about my marriage. People can be really judgmental sometimes! My husband is a card shark. He also plays golf. I have never given him a hard time about his hobbies because every second that he is home he is Super-Dad—fully engaged with me and the kids. I have no desire to play cards or golf. Our hobbies are different on purpose. This is part of the "secret sauce" of our marriage. Every marriage is unique and works with different parameters, but this is the truth about mine. He needs time to be with friends and unwind without me and the kids, and I need that, too. He jokes that the day I take up golf is the day he quits—and I agree!

The comments I hear fluctuate between "You're nuts," and "You're wife of the year." But I simply think that the time we spend apart makes the time we are together better. I am not saying this is how it is or should be for everyone. I am only telling you what works for us. I don't begrudge his time away because in turn it gives me the freedom to say that I want to take a yoga class or walk with a friend when I need some down time. It works both ways in my house. And it works like this with pretty much everyone in my life. I adore being around those I care about, and then I need a bit of time to regroup by myself. That is why my self-care routines are non-negotiables for me.

When I think about what helps me get the most out of motherhood, it is the combination of spending time with my kids where I am truly present and engaged, balanced with having time to refuel and fill my own cup. I practice meditation, I journal, I pray, I exercise, I read, and I dream a lot. These all in turn make me a way better mom. I know it. My husband knows it. My kids know it. I also spend a lot of time with my dogs. There are days that I could get a ton more done, but I stop between every task for big-time puppy snuggles. Some days I wish more than anything my dogs could talk to me, and others, when things are hectic or the kids are being whiny, I am so glad that they can't!

I have also discovered along my journey of being a mom that I can refuel by being near my family while simultaneously having quiet time. This happens when we engage in an activity like reading, where we are near each other but aren't necessarily interacting. I actually love these times! I can look over at my kids and marvel at their features, offer a smile, and go back to my book. I have been a bookworm since college, and the first time that I was on the couch with both of my kids, and we were all three reading silently,

I actually cried! I had literally dreamt of that day where I could share one of my favorite pastimes with my kids. They thought I was such a dork!

We can start working with our kids so that these quiet times, or breaks, are a natural part of the rhythm of the household. Independent play is an important skill, and I learned this firsthand by seeing the differences in my son who got more independent play time because he was the second.

With my firstborn I was attentive every single second, playing on the floor for hours and watching every minute thing he did. Even as a preteen he still wants me to watch every dive into the pool. I had chilled out a bit with my second, and I gave him more independent play time. He is happy when I watch and happy when I don't.

Independent play is a fundamental component in a child's growth. When kids play independently they use their imagination, which can help them be more successful in life. Watching television doesn't count as independent play! Think along the lines of playing with dolls or cars, coloring, playing make-believe, or building with Legos. Even as kids get a bit older, they can still play like this. My boys have baseball cards and small plastic football helmets, and they can play with them for hours. Magnatiles also offer tons of longevity, even as kids get older. (If you don't have Magnatiles, they are completely worth the investment. They are transparent, flat magnetic blocks that you can build with on the floor or in 3D.) I have had five ten-year-olds building with Magnatiles for an entire afternoon, and they are amazing for boys and girls.

Playtime needs to be balanced just like anything in life. Your kids need to play with you, and they need to play by themselves. The time that our kids are playing independently can be used for self-care, chores, Sunday meal prep, or organizing your desk. You could

also sit down with your spouse and do that thing that you never get to do. Not *that* thing, but you can actually have a conversation.

I have always meditated in the early mornings, but occasionally my kids get up super early and come downstairs. I have had to train them that I cannot be interrupted during my practice unless there is an emergency. I have always welcomed my kids into my "zen den" and have invited them to sit quietly near me, meditate along with me, or read quietly. They were never turned away as long as they were quiet. If they are in the mood to snuggle I have let them lay their head on my lap as I meditate, but everyone has a different tolerance for distraction. I am never one to turn away a snuggle!

This was a perfect opportunity to teach the kids about respect for someone's practices and space. Until my kids were in school full time, almost every minute of my day-to-day life revolved around my kids' needs, except these few precious minutes, and I deserved that time. Frankly, I came to depend on it for the rest of the day to run smoothly! There is nothing wrong with having boundaries and asking your kids to respect them. I think it is an important life lesson that will help them when they live with roommates, and even spouses one day.

Now that my kids are growing up, I am having to learn to respect their boundaries as well. Occasionally they need down time away from me, and even when I ask them to play cards or take the dogs on a walk, they don't always want to. At first my feelings got hurt, but I opened myself up to the lesson for me as a mom. If I need personal time and space each day, why should it be any different for them? I realized that it wasn't about me; they were simply learning and growing into their own and gaining the awareness of what feels right to them and when. Isn't this what I want? It took some adjusting to not have everything be on my terms, but in this

case my children became wonderful teachers for me. *It isn't all about me.*

A dialogue began to open up when I created a safe space for the kids to tell me what they needed from me. Was it a hug, conversation, or space?

They realized that they could share their feelings with me without worrying about hurting mine. Our lines of communication have stayed so open because I don't force them to talk when they aren't in the mood. I have realized that my younger son likes to open up after school, and my older son likes to open up when I am tucking him in at night. I don't push him to give me details earlier in the day because I know his habits and that he most likely will open up before bed. This has helped me to relax and understand that he isn't shutting me out; I just need to be patient.

Some kids like to open up in the car, before bed, on the way to school, or after school. Some like to share with their friends around, and others tend to be more private. Simply begin to become aware of your child's patterns and comfort levels, and I suspect you won't feel like you have to push quite so hard.

Conclusion

One of my very favorite inspiring mom quotes is from Jodi Picoult. She states that, "The very fact that you care about being a good mom means that you already are one." I couldn't agree more. And that means *you*! That's right: you are amazing!

You picked up this book because something about the title *Get the Most Out of Motherhood* intrigued you. You wanted the tips and tools to make that happen. We have covered a ton of ground over these chapters together, so now what?

I beg of you not to make this book the equivalent of buying a gym membership on January first and ditching it by March. Utilizing the tools in this book is part of your journey. Change takes time, and remember, baby steps totally count!

Go slow! Motherhood is not a race. Using these tools should not add to your stress. These tools are your way out—if you practice them. I simply beg of you to practice them with self-compassion at the forefront of your mind.

Trust me, you will make progress, fall off the wagon, and repeat that cycle again. Let go of any guilt you usually pile on, and simply

start where you left off. You can do it! I believe in you with every ounce of me.

It is impossible to think that you will take thirty-one tidbits and simultaneously weave them into the fabric of your life. Trying to do too much too fast won't lead to long-term success and solidifying new habits.

My very best advice, and you know that I wouldn't steer you wrong, is to pick one or two tools that really speak to you and start there. I promise even one small tweak or change in your stale routine can make a mountain of difference. You will feel re-energized and motivated to be the mom you are meant to be.

When one tweak has turned into a routine that feels good, in-corporate another tweak into your routine. Pause and begin again at your own pace. Follow your intuition and feel free to use my sug-gestions as a starting point and make them your own as you see fit.

I've shared my experience as a mom—how I bond and connect with my own kids—all while being honest about the struggle and mistakes I have made along my journey thus far. If you have ever felt alone in parenting, I hope this book has changed that, and you have the tools you need to get the most out of motherhood. By sharing so candidly and openly, I hope to have given you motivation, and per-mission if that is what you feel you need, to admit that motherhood can feel like the best job in the world some days, and a complete struggle on others. You aren't doing anything wrong! If you ever have days where you wonder, "Is this what it's supposed to be like and feel like?" I totally do, too! If you wonder if you are screwing up, the answer is yes, but rest assured you are in really good company. Why do you think I have so much good advice to share? I have made a lot of mistakes—and learned from them! My contribution to this world is helping other moms to be better from everything I have learned.

If you feel as if you gained even one tool to make your life as a mom better, or gathered a bit of wisdom for how to bond with your kids, then I have done my job. I am going to go out on a limb and say I hope you got that and then some!

Use me. That's right, I am giving you permission to use me! I hope that you do utilize me beyond this book. I have so many ways that you can take advantage of me, and many of them are free.

- Sign up for my weekly newsletter at www.hotmesstomindfulmom.com. It is filled with inspiration and motivation around self-care and mindful parenting.
- Join the amazing community of like-minded moms in my Facebook Group by searching "Hot Mess to Mindful Mom Community" on Facebook. The vibe is low-key, authentic, and supportive.
- Join the party on Instagram: @alikatz_hotmesstomindfulmom.
- Try my FREE guided meditation challenge at www.hotmesstomindfulmom.com.

Celebrate that you have read this book from start to finish and you are gaining tools and a better understanding of how to help yourself and your family make the most of this one beautiful life. I am honored to have been on this journey with you. **XO**

Acknowledgments

My family and friends have been an amazing support during the writing of "book 2" and knowing that they are behind me makes every project even more fun.

My clients and students let me live my purpose and passion, and I am grateful for everyone in the *Hot Mess to Mindful Mom* Community.

Mark, Adam, and Dylan, there are no words for how much I love you, and how much your support means to me.

To my editor, Leah Zarra, you have helped bring my words to life, and made my ideas shine. I feel truly fortunate to have your support and the pleasure of working with Skyhorse Publishing.

About the Author

Ali Katz is a self-care and mindful parenting coach, a meditation teacher, and a motivational speaker. Ali lives in Houston, Texas, but works with women all over the world. When not writing or coaching, Ali enjoys spending time with her family, sipping tea, and snuggling with her dogs.

You can learn more about Ali and her private and group coaching programs and meditation classes at www.hotmesstomindfulmom .com.

If you are looking for a community of like-minded moms, consider joining Ali's Facebook group at www.facebook.com/groups /hotmesstomindfulmomcommunity.